MEMORY

Memory: Shaping Connections in the Arts Therapies is a compilation of scholarly chapters by authors of global reputation in the arts therapies.

This international publication reflects the theme of the 16th International Conference of the European Consortium for Arts Therapies (ECArTE), held in Vilnius, Lithuania. Questions of memory go to the very heart of our making sense of the world. This book brings together wide-ranging chapters which address the question of memory, designed to stimulate understanding and debate in contemporary arts therapy education, practice and research.

Writers from Canada, Estonia, Germany, Iceland, Lebanon, Lithuania, Spain, the UK and US combine to create a topical publication, incorporating diverse and current thinking in art therapy, dance movement therapy, dramatherapy and music therapy. In this innovative compilation, authors offer different cultural perspectives on the conception of memory which informs epistemology across the field of arts therapy.

This book will be of interest and relevance to those in the arts therapy community and to a broader readership, including students and professionals in the disciplines of psychology, sociology, psychotherapy, the arts, medicine, integrated health and education.

Marián Cao is an Art Therapist and Professor of Art Education and Art Therapy at the University Complutense of Madrid, Spain. She teaches and lectures in Spain and internationally. Founder director of the Arts Therapy Masters' programme at University Complutense of Madrid, and former director of the PhD programme on Art, Art Therapy and Social Inclusion, she has coordinated several Latinoamerican University programmes.

Richard Hougham is a Principal Lecturer at the Royal Central School of Speech and Drama, University of London, where he is course leader for the MA Drama and Movement Therapy programme. He is currently Chair of the Executive Board of the European Consortium for Arts Therapies Education (ECArTE) and has a particular interest in intercultural dialogues and epistemology in the international teaching of arts therapies.

Sarah Scoble is Honorary President of ECArTE. She served on the Executive Board of ECArTE for many years and was Chair from 2009 to 2017. Founder trainer in south west UK in Dramatherapy and former director of Masters in Dramatherapy programmes, University of Exeter, she is Series Editor with Diane Waller for an annual *International Research in the Arts Therapies* publication with Routledge, in association with ECArTE and the International Centre for Research in Arts Therapies (ICRA).

This volume follows a series of eleven previous books, all inspired by and emerging from ECArTE's biennial international conferences.

This is ECArTE's second such publication with Routledge.

MEMORY

Shaping Connections in the Arts Therapies

Edited by Marián Cao, Richard Hougham, Sarah Scoble

Routledge
Taylor & Francis Group
LONDON AND NEW YORK

ECArTE
EUROPEAN CONSORTIUM FOR ARTS THERAPIES EDUCATION

Cover image: *The (Mis)adventures of Pinocchio.* © Photograph Melissa Castillo Molina, 2022.

First published 2025
by Routledge
4 Park Square, Milton Park, Abingdon, Oxon OX14 4RN

and by Routledge
605 Third Avenue, New York, NY 10158

Routledge is an imprint of the Taylor & Francis Group, an informa business

British Library Cataloguing-in-Publication Data
A catalogue record for this book is available from the British Library

ISBN: 978-1-032-66817-8 (hbk)
ISBN: 978-1-032-66819-2 (pbk)
ISBN: 978-1-032-66394-4 (ebk)

DOI: 10.4324/9781032663944

Typeset in Times New Roman
by Apex CoVantage, LLC

In memory of Dr Dorothy Langley

EUROPEAN CONSORTIUM FOR ARTS THERAPIES EDUCATION (ECArTE)

The European Consortium for Arts Therapies Education was founded in 1991. It is a non-profit-making organisation, which was established with the support of ERASMUS. ECArTE is a consortium of universities. Its primary purpose is to represent and encourage the development of arts therapies and arts therapies education in Europe; in particular, the courses offering nationally validated and professionally recognised training for arts therapists. (The Arts Therapies include art therapy, dance therapy, dramatherapy, play therapy and music therapy).

The Universities of Hertfordshire, Münster, Nijmegen and Paris founded ECArTE in 1991. Currently, it comprises 34 member institutions from 13 European countries.

The consortium's work includes:

- Creating stronger European links in the Arts Therapies through the international exchange of staff and students.
- Promoting research into methods of Arts Therapies practice within Europe.
- Working towards opportunities for international study and exchange in Arts Therapies training programmes.
- Promoting recognition of qualifications in Arts Therapies at a European level.
- Supporting the development of appropriate, academically recognised, nationally validated Higher Education courses for the Arts Therapies.
- Publishing academic texts on current practices, philosophies and research in international Arts Therapies.
- Offering opportunities for professional communication and development at its international conferences.
- Working towards mutual collaboration in all aspects of Arts Therapies development and practice across Europe.
- Supporting the design, development and validation of new programmes in all member states.
- Communicating with policy and strategic departments to educate and inform them about the discipline of the Arts Therapies.

European Network

ECArTE is working towards establishing mutual recognition and compatibility in educational and vocational training for arts therapists within the European Community. The criteria for membership to ECArTE are subject to a changing educational and social landscape. There are complex articulations of qualifications in different European Countries and ECArTE is keen to remain observant of these differences and inclusive in its practice.

CONTENTS

LIST OF FIGURES

Cover image: *The (Mis)adventures of Pinocchio*. © Photograph Melissa Castillo Molina, 2022.

This photograph was taken from a performance during the conference – 'The (Mis)adventures of Pinocchio and the Unreliable Shapeshifter, OR: From Senex to Senility and Back Again'.

This was a collaboration between artists, arts therapists and students, which explored aspects of autobiographical memory and invited the audience to enter into the mind of Pinocchio in his old age.

PREFACE

This book is the 12th in a series of ECArTE conference publications. It is a compilation of some of the inspirational and innovative work presented in Vilnius, Lithuania, in 2022. One of the hallmarks of the ECArTE conferences is an endeavour to listen and respond to the *genius loci* of the place. In other words, to listen to its spirit and history and ask how this might influence the theme of the conference itself. Vilnius is a city of cultural and artistic depth, heritage and complexity. The theme of "memory" was born out of the stirring feelings that Vilnius carries within its people, buildings and art and how as a community of arts therapists we might engage with and reflect on these reverberations. Questions of memory go to the very heart of our making sense of the world, in terms of a capacity for reflection, whether bidden or unbidden. Plato's original epistemology presented memory as a recollection of an inherited knowledge. A kind of storehouse of the soul. In an example of curious conflation, Plato's classical idea of *anamnesis*, which described a calling to mind of a previous existence, is now language in contemporary psychiatry for a case history of a psychiatric patient. Such echoes of language and ideas abound in psychoanalysis and the development of psychotherapy has been informed and shaped by these philosophical roots.

Important questions seemed to emerge from these roots. For example, how does art shape our collective memory of the past and how might it inform our experience of major events in our own time? Artists use the arts to tell stories about personal and cultural memory that are open to interpretation, reframing the past not as a fixed narrative but as a multiplicity of voices from diverse points of view. This allows us to think twice about our history, how it has been shaped and how we might best document things to come. The arts have, historically, offered a means for memories to move away from literal narrative, or positivist tropes, into symbolic and aesthetic forms. This opens up the opportunity for investigation of memories as artefacts, materials and spaces which contain and elicit stories of the past, present and future. It invites a performative rendering of memory in its many forms. The arts can move memory away from sequential time and causality, asking how memories present and reveal themselves. Through the body, memory captures attention in the senses, kindling a recollection through a momentary assemblage of impressions or the capacity to remember songs and music even when cognition is impaired. Memories are sometimes written, but they are also transmitted, in movements, dreams, paintings, sounds and music.

Memory can also be cast as memorial and an act of remembrance. There are rituals, markers and symbolic moments of performance, which trace events from the past and remember the ancestors. Different cosmologies and religions employ performance practices, artefacts and storytelling as ways to honour memories and engage kinaesthetically and ritually. And what of the forgettings? The capsules of time and experience which have been lost and are waiting in the wings to be recalled. Psychologically, there are the problems of individual and collective repression, distortion and denial, along with the well-documented consequences of such psychodynamic processes. The ways in which the arts link with such psychoanalytical ideas offer many routes for enquiry, such as Freud's notion of "afterwardsness" (Nachträglichkeit), the nature of dissociation and questions of trans-generational trauma. In analytical psychology, there is the research carried out by Jung into cultural memory, leading to his formulation of the collective unconscious as an ancestral or inherited memory observed through dreams and the cultural narratives of myth and story. There is also contemporary research into memory in the fields of neurology, neurobiology and neuroscience, disciplines that are increasingly collaborating with the arts. Questions of how sensations, physical actions and artistic practices (e.g. singing, dancing, painting and sculpting) evoke and elicit memory have inspired multiple interdisciplinary projects which reflect neuroscientific research, which connects with the arts. How such questions of memory connect with the arts therapies seemed to be a galvanising and productive theme for a conference, which generated some excellent presentations, workshops and performances. This volume is a selection of contributions which present an international set of authors and representation from the different arts therapy modalities.

The opening chapter by Nisha Sajnani from her keynote at the conference and addresses central concerns of cultural memory and its temporality. Initially examining the place of metaphor and symbol in the arts therapies, she moves on to direct our attention to monuments and how we experience memory in the public sphere. Questions of what such memorials and representations hold for people and symbolise are examined critically, alongside questions of what knowledge arts therapies consider and teach, in light of contested histories and questionable beliefs and actions.

Audronė Brazauskaitė presents an anthropological approach to the symbolic meaning of knots and their relation to memory. Taking a journey through ancient cultures, she explores what weaving, knotting, plaiting and untying symbolise and articulates a discourse that relates the mythopoetic metaphors of textile artefacts to the most prominent metaphors of life – destiny, time, path, sacrifice and binding. From this theoretical incursion, Brazauskaitė proposes an art therapeutic process in which knots are metaphors related to life, and tactile experiences encourage sensory stimulation and implicit memory.

Gabriele Schmid reflects in her chapter on embodied memory and the capacity of animals to share states of fear and other emotions, relevant in the artworks she analyses: the Belgian artist Berlinde De Bruyckere, the American artist Matthew Barney, the Lithuanian artist Eglė Budvytytė and the Ukrainian artist and co-founder of Femen, Oksana Shachko. The interrelation of the human and non-human world is present in her text. Schmid cites concepts of Margulis that dissolve the dichotomies that have characterised Western thought. For example, in considering life as cyclical and by examining the organic phenomenon of symbiosis, the author proposes new and innovative ideas for art therapy.

There is another rendition of different types of memory in the chapter by Marián Cao as she refers to exemplary and literal memory as explored by Tzvetan Todorov. In this chapter, Cao proffers a different attention, one which draws on the ancient Greek idea of the Aedo, an artist who sang epics which drew on collective experience and – as Cao suggests "collected the strands of the memory of pain and recomposed them". We are presented with an exposition rich in context and cultural artistic practices, as we read and imagine the work of the three contemporary artists and collectives – Doris Salcedo, Gustavo Germano and Art al Quadrat. This chapter brings memory into the senses, into materiality and elegantly draws us into memory as somehow tangible, like the sand, stone and water in Salcedo's piece "When the Stone Cries" or the physical sensation and enactment of shaving heads in the piece by the art collective Art al Quadrat. Central to Cao's work is a philosophical examination of associated themes which reside in the very notion of memory, such as absence, forgetting and forgiveness.

Vera Heller offers a striking example of how autoethnographic research based on the arts stands as a privileged means of narrating oneself in relation to the past and the cultural context and can be a powerful tool in art therapy. Using the first person, the chapter delicately threads text and images, opening access to individual and collective memory. In this way, it brings the reader into the present through an autoethnography that has been developed over three years. The self-narrative becomes a tool for transformation, reconstructing the past from the present and helping to reconfigure identity and transform traumatic memories into a "permanent memorial". Heller relates her proposal to three artists – Antony Tàpies, Louise Bourgeois and Anselm Kiefer – all of whom have constantly evoked memory in their work.

Joy Gravestock's groundbreaking chapter explores her hypothesis, developed over recent years, that music therapy can provide a way for adoptee and therapist to become aware together of the client's previously unrepresented experience and embodied memory. She takes us deep into questions of memory with skill and compassion and argues persuasively that, through music therapy, adoption-specific memory when recovered, witnessed and held safely can become "memory reframed and repaired". Drawing on Stern's affective attunement, Reich's understanding of the pre-linguistic nature of emotional experience and expression, Freud's *après-coup* and the notion of Plato's anamnesis, she weaves together critical discussion and clinical vignettes in a beautifully crafted and affecting narrative.

In a carefully balanced chapter, Alanah Garrard combines theory and clinical examples to explore and analyse ways in which dramatherapy can work with autobiographical memory. In particular, it illuminates ways in which the dramatherapist's use of movement, play and story can stimulate the discovery of new perspectives on personal myth and memory. Rooted in contemporary theory and influenced by the philosophy of Merleau-Ponty, Sartre and Heidegger, Garrard takes a phenomenological stance in the practice of dramatherapy to elucidate, examine and address the sense of self. The reader is invited to consider how personal myths, formed through childhood or through memories, stories and perspectives of others, might be loosened and reframed. Her emphasis is away from cognitive retelling, enabling the body's felt understanding of experience to be known through movement and so opens the opportunity for change. The chapter immerses us thoughtfully in deliberations on the making and breaking of personal myth.

The chapter by Unnur Óttarsdóttir focuses her research on children who have suffered trauma. It explores how emotions which relate to difficult events in the child's life that have not been processed, integrated, and worked through affect the child's emotional well-being and school learning. Her intervention focuses on how the intersection of emotions linked to stress and trauma can be managed effectively through art therapy and, at the same time, improve retention of academic material through drawing. The aim of the research, through grounded theory, is to create, analyse and validate a therapeutic approach aimed at promoting emotional well-being and academic understanding in children dealing with the aftermath of stress, trauma and specific learning challenges.

In a compelling study, Sara Sakhi, Farah Wardani, Lina Kreidie, Karima Anbar and HH Sheikha Intisar Al Sabah movingly explore their work with a group of refugee women in Lebanon. Together they examine the role of dramatherapy in revisiting and honouring the shadows of war in the women. In a frank and poignant account, the chapter examines the progress and impact of a dramatherapy programme, which took place in Shatila camp. The sessions were designed to create a sacred space in which to work with the "festering invisible wounds" of some of the millions of women affected by war in the Arab world. The author-practitioners apply a reflexive duo-ethnographic approach to revisit their own memories and experiences of working with the women and the themes which surfaced of dispossession, loss, fragility, pain, grief, deprivation, marginalisation, "the resilience of helplessness", survival and hope. The programme resulted in a play, based on the participants' personal stories, extracts from which the women have kindly given their permission to share in this publication.

Eha Rüütel and Raquel Stephenson introduce research carried out in Estonia, called the "Dementia Project", in which new creative arts therapists were trained with the necessary skills to work with older people with dementia. Based on how the arts and art therapy can be a way of working with older dementia patients, improving cognitive capacity, psychological well-being, lifestyle and sense of personhood again, the three-phase programme prepares students to approach this scenario by developing their abilities and resources. The training offered an immersive learning experience, shedding light on various crucial facets of the distinctive characteristics and difficulties that emerging practitioners encounter in their engagements with elderly individuals grappling with dementia.

The final chapter is a transcription of an interview with Aleka Loutsis, who offers fascinating ideas about the notion of memory in dramatherapy and dance movement therapy. The conversation, though improvised, seems to return to the central theme of implicit and explicit memory. The question of implicit memory is discussed as a more mysterious and irrational phenomenon and extrapolated through dialogue and examples. Explicit memory is considered as memory which is available to recall and bring into consciousness at will. What is compelling in this conversation is the relationship between the two: the explicit and the implicit. It elucidates convincingly how drama and movement therapy can offer ways to connect with and give form to these different types of memory. Loutsis also brings our attention to the ways in which memory is held in the body and offers insights into how the developmental gestures of yielding, pushing, reaching, grasping and pulling can be adopted in the practice of the arts therapies.

The combination and diversity of these chapters demonstrate the complexity and philosophical depth of the theme. The authors have taken the theme of memory into new and original territory, drawing from art history, contemporary art, psychoanalysis and philosophy. Such a breadth of mapping reflects the emerging potential of arts therapy theory and practice, as it shapes its epistemology and research through interdisciplinary dialogue.

The Editors
Marián Cao, Richard Hougham, Sarah Scoble
2024

ACKNOWLEDGEMENTS

The editors would like to thank Laura Hussey for her tireless enthusiasm and positive support through the development of this publication. Additionally, we extend our grateful thanks to Swatti Hindwan and Nick Craggs for their efficiency and helpfulness as we worked with them through the publication processes. Our thanks, too, to members of the local organising committee in Vilnius for their assistance in the organisation of ECArTE's 16th international conference.

A special thanks to Matthew Gammage for his generous and reliable contribution to this publication as our proofreader. And, of course, we extend our sincere thanks to the diligent authors, all of whom have shared their knowledge, skills and expertise to make this publication possible and to build the body of knowledge in the arts therapies.

1

MOSS, MEMORY AND THE CONTRADICTORY IMAGINATION

Nisha Sajnani

Abstract

This chapter is based on my keynote address for the 16th conference of the European Consortium for Arts Therapies Education (ECArTE)[1]. Drawing on examples of current negotiations of public monuments in post-Soviet Vilnius and other sites, I discuss the role of symbols and metaphors in facilitating our capacities to attend to contradictions in private and cultural memory.

Keywords: metaphor, symbols, memory, decolonisation, Lithuania, politics, creative arts therapies

Introduction

Given its current and historical negotiation of public streets and monuments, the post-Soviet capital of Lithuania, Vilnius, provided an ideal context for the 16th conference of the European Consortium for Arts Therapies Education (ECArTE) focused on the theme of memory. Drawing on my keynote address for this convening, I begin with a personal and political perspective for a discussion of symbols and metaphors with regard to attending to memory in the creative arts therapies. Then, drawing on examples from Vilnius and elsewhere, I explore the pivotal role of symbols and metaphors in facilitating our capacities to attend to contradictions in private and public spaces.

Personal and political context

My original keynote was delivered a few days after the death of Queen Elizabeth II, the longest-reigning monarch in the UK, having ruled for seventy years. In

DOI: 10.4324/9781032663944-1

India, the country of my parents' birth prior to Partition in 1947, the memories of British rule marked by the subjugation of the people of then-undivided India were fresh in public memory when Elizabeth II ascended to the throne in 1952, a mere five years later. In a personal recording, I captured historian Rana Safvi recalling her early memories of seeing the Queen for the first time. Her words offer evidence of the power of symbols and the contradictions that we may inhabit in times like these.

> Growing up in those days, on fairy tales, a queen was a magical figure . . . it was the first time we had seen a queen. I have very clear memories of her dress. It was a blue dress, and I remember the guards on horses. Today when we see it, we don't see it just with a lot of you know, romantic sentiments of a queen or a royal family. Today, we also see it as part of the exploitation of the colonies and imperialism . . . but condoling the death of a queen who embodied dignity and even duty in her life does not mean that you're condoning colonialism or imperialism[2].

Her words convey the negotiation of memory circulating between powerful impressions left from childhood fairy tales, the emotional weight encoded during the rich symbolic pageantry of a royal visit and an adult's awareness of the impact of colonial rule. Safvi's words convey her psychological capacity to hold duality, a capacity that many people who have suffered oppression have had to master to survive when she speaks about acknowledging the dignity and duty of the individual woman who played the role of Queen and the colonial exploitation represented by British imperialism. This kind of pluralism is something we may struggle with in our private lives and in the public sphere where the voices of many are often subjugated to the choices of the few with the social, financial, military, religious, technological or legal means to enforce their version of the truth, and its material consequences, in an increasingly post-truth reality. As the playwright James Baldwin (1961) said of the criminal systemic indifference towards violence against Black people in America, where I recently became – after years of ambivalence – a citizen, "to be a Negro in this country and to be relatively conscious is to be in a state of rage almost, almost all of the time". One is trained to dissociate, to live in the interstices of what W.E.B. Du Bois (2008) called a "double consciousness" to refer to the struggle that African Americans may face to remain true to Black culture while at the same time conforming to a dominant white society to survive. This chapter is about the role of symbols and metaphors in revealing the complexity of this paradox and its influence on the shaping of memory and our possible futures.

Symbols, metaphors and the embrace of contradiction in the creative arts therapies

One of the great benefits of the creative arts therapies is that they do not rely on verbal or literal language alone. We use the arts as a way of talking and as a space of refuge within a therapeutic relationship. The uses of symbols and metaphors have been much discussed across the creative arts therapies (see Eberhard-Kaechele, 2012; Hougham & Jones, 2017; Leite, 2003; Mann, 1996; Moon, 2007; Smeijsters, 2012) and were recently identified as being amongst the most salient therapeutic factors that are shared across modalities of practice (deWitte, *et al*, 2021).

Symbols act as a bridge between the conscious and unconscious imagination. In the context of therapy, symbolisation through colour, form, movement, sound, lyrics, characters, costumes and props, for example, enables contact with and facilitates the representation of one's inner world in ways that may be beneficial for well-being. The stroke of a paintbrush or physical gesture may not be entirely decoupled from the social and cultural contexts that give them meaning or render them legible to others but may, for a time, suspend the need to immediately extract reason and meaning in favour of enabling the exploration of multiple and, at times, contradictory meanings. Drama therapists Ramsden and Landy (2021) describe the necessity of accepting contradiction and paradox:

> Human beings strive toward balance and harmony, and although they never fully arrive, they have the capacity to accept the consequences of living with contradiction and paradox. It is not ultimately the need to resolve cognitive dissonance that motivates human behaviour, but rather the need to live with paradox.
>
> *(p. 85)*

In a similar way, metaphors, which transfer something from one context and place it in a different context to produce new understanding, hold information that hides meaning in symbolic form (Draaisma, 2000). Törneke (2010) writes that "metaphoric language transfers functions from one experiential field to another", which is what gives symbols and metaphors enormous power in psychotherapy (p. 10). Metaphors provide the transfer of something someone already knows and is convinced of to a new situation which can facilitate insight and self-discovery. In order to be most effective, symbols and metaphors must be culturally relevant. In order to extract new meaning from the phrase "time is a river", for example, one needs to know what a river is.

The use of metaphors has also been taken up in general psychotherapies as an effective way for individuals and groups to make sense of themselves and their environments in a world that is excessively structured by literal language. Over the last few decades, research on metaphors, in particular, has demonstrated that they are not only rhetorical devices but are, in fact, culturally conditioned and fundamental to how we understand concepts, structure knowledge, remember the past, experience the present and imagine the future. Metaphors create what Sapolsky (2010) has referred to as "neural confusion" wherein our brains treat literal and metaphoric language in the same way. Psychologists Thibodeau and Boroditsky (2011) conducted a study which indicated that even the subtlest utterance of a metaphor, via a single word, can have a powerful influence over how we attempt to solve pressing concerns and how we gather information to make decisions. They also found that the influence of the metaphorical framing effect is covert: people do not recognise metaphors as influential in the way they recall information or make decisions. Taken together, symbols and metaphors hold enormous influence over what is encoded, suppressed and surfaced in memory and this influence can be seen in public cultural practice.

Memory wars in public spaces in Vilnius

There are several examples of this phenomenon in Vilnius where, at the time of writing, symbols of public and private recollection were being debated in real-time. Russia's aggressive war in Ukraine unleashed a wave of initiatives across Lithuania to remove the remaining signs of its Soviet past. The Lithuanian parliament recently drafted a "desovietisation" bill in order to speed up not only the removal of statues and monuments but to also change the remaining names of streets and squares that are reminders of Soviet occupation. As Paulė Kuzmickienė, the chair of the Commission for Freedom Struggles and Historical Memory in Lithuania, stated, "it is very important . . . to discuss who were the people after whom streets are named, what they mean for our state and our history" (Lisauskaitė, 2022). These memory wars call up recent attempts to rid the US landscape of monuments to the Confederacy following nationwide protests against systemic racism and its many manifestations (Cohen, 2017).

Yet, some have raised concerns about these acts of erasure – the erasing of physical traces of violence, occupation, and colonial history for fear that the suppression or loss of these symbolic markers may result in the repetition of violence. They point to the value and psychological necessity of symbolic representation. In one instance, Matthew Moore, an American artist-in-residence at the Vilnius Academy of Art, asked, "Where do these statues go?" What do we do with the undesirable, the unpreferred? What is left in their absence? In his photo documentation of places where monuments once stood, Moore (2020) wrote:

> These photographs seem to portray obscure public squares or city parks, but to some local inhabitants, these spaces are charged with a more ominous presence. In some cases, the absence of the statue is more obvious, while in others the local government has gone to great lengths to transform the space.

In another instance of art and the transformation of social memory, Lithuanian artists Eglė Grėbliauskaitė and Agnė Gintalaitė were given permission by Vilnius City authorities, to respond to a statue of the writer Petras Cvirka, which had become a flashpoint on the question of whether to preserve these remaining monuments of an era long gone or preserve the few that remain as symbols of remembrance and healing. Critics said his dissemination of pro-Soviet propaganda, and his role in denouncing his contemporaries, made him unsuitable for public reverence, as well as an affront to victims of the Soviet regime. Yet others pointed out that while Cvirka's pro-Soviet actions are well-documented, his works remained an important part of Lithuania's cultural canon. They asked, "If Cvirka's statue is removed then which monument will be next to follow?" (Nielsen, 2021).

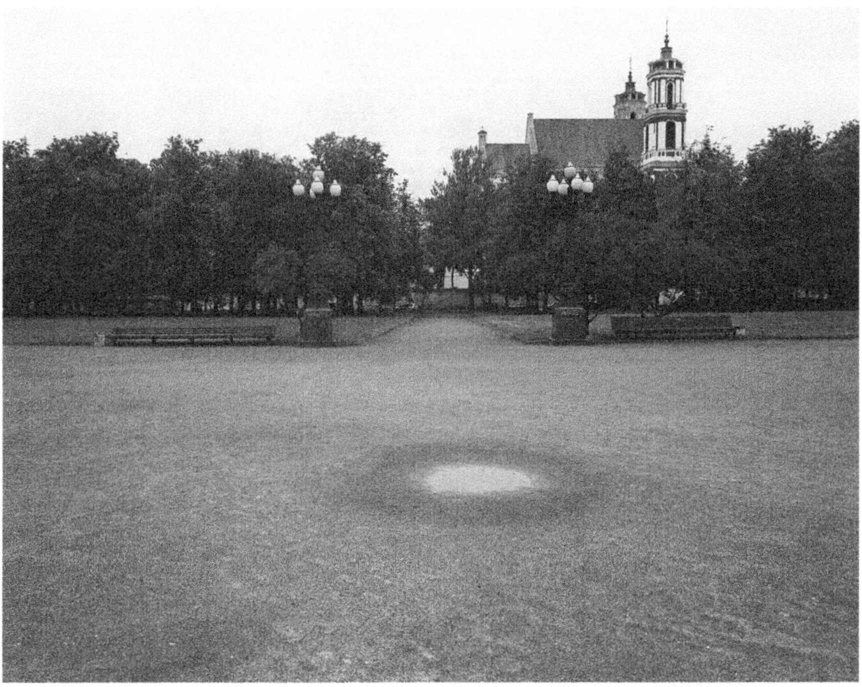

FIGURE 1.1 Lenin, Vilnius, Lithuania, 2014. Credit: Matthew Moore.

These artists sought a third path of dealing with the modern politics of public memory through another symbol of healing and transformation – Lithuanian moss – which they used to drape the statue in an installation they called *Let's Not Forget Not to Remember*. Grėbliauskaitė stated:

> Moss, as a symbol of time and healing, capitalizes on nature's capacity to heal the trauma of occupation and colonialism that is so urgent in today's society . . . The strategy could be used as a solution not only to Soviet-era monuments, but also with statues [linked to] colonialism. Moss covers up the glorification of ideology, but still preserves history.
>
> *(Grėbliauskaitė in Nielsen, 2021)*

Yet, as the art installation was unfolding, officials seemed to have a change of heart. The presence of this statue, however transformed, was still intolerable to some. The licence for the art project was revoked and the artists were ordered to halt their work, leading to the removal of the statue on November 19, 2021.

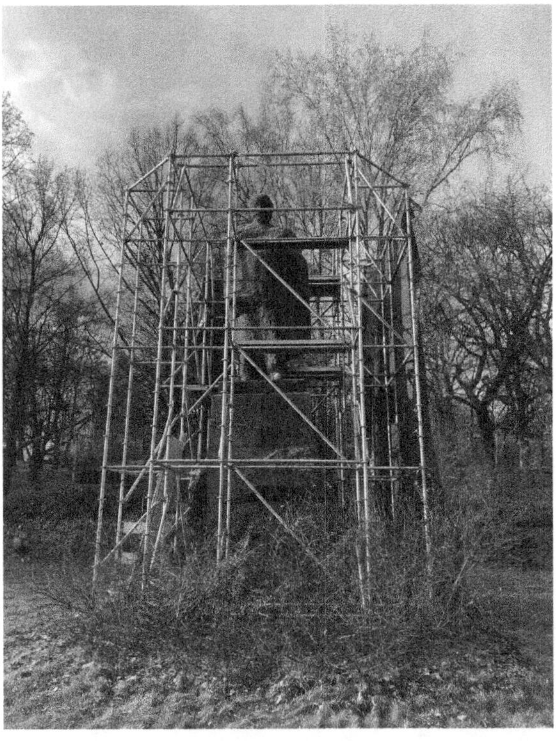

FIGURE 1.2 *Let's Not Forget Not to Remember*, 2021. Credit: Eglė Grėbliauskaitė and Agnė Gintalaitė.

Negotiating monument(al) figures in the creative arts therapies

In *Civilization and its Discontents*, Freud (1930) imagined memory as Rome, a city built upon the layers and layers of past cities going all the way back to the Palatine Hill. So do the missing and contradictory voices that populate contemporary struggles for memory layer upon each other in our individual and collective bodies, summoned to the surface as an exercise of power, by choice or as unbidden echoes resounding through the repetition of history and our anticipated futures. A major difference, of course, is that our work, in the creative arts therapies, seldom takes the form of immovable statues that endure over decades, though we might consider how the foundations of our field function to preserve grand narratives that may seem just as solid.

Consider the controversies that surround Rudolph Laban's affiliation with the Third Reich. Laban, an early founder of European modern dance whose approach to movement analysis is widely taught in dance movement therapy and has informed other arts therapies (Fernandes, 2016; Young & Wood, 2018), thrived under Nazi rule (Dickson, 2016). Yet, as Dickson wrote, there is ambivalence about how to hold competing narratives about his contributions.

> Many historians who have researched Laban's career either brush by the fact that he worked for the Nazis or portray him as having been forced to do so. Interpretations about Laban's participation in Nazism vary widely and, though many consider Laban to be a victim of coercion, a less popular but perhaps more feasible explanation is that Laban voluntarily chose to align himself with the Third Reich.
>
> *(p. 1)*

How have we, in the creative arts therapies, grappled with this history? Should Laban be removed from dance movement therapy training as Cvirka's statue was? Is there an equivalent to Lithuanian moss that might offer a third way to contend with these complicated shadows and alternate histories? Should there be? Can moss lead to meaningful repair and reparations? To justice?

Not all examples are as dramatic. What of the myths chosen in drama therapy? Safvi's memories of the influence of fairy tales in shaping her imagination, the normalisation of monarchy, and her internalised subjectivity, underscore the critical and always already political, choices made in our practice. How do we remember those voices that may, for one reason or another, be suppressed or silenced in the work that we do where ephemeral traces of intergenerational, collective and individual memory appear and disappear in clay, paper, sound, gestures, roles, stories and scenes? (Dokter and Sajnani, 2023).

Conclusion

This chapter is an investigation of the role of symbols and metaphors in facilitating our personal and collective capacities to attend to the complexity and contradiction in private and cultural memory– and the limits of the same. We are in a period of great transformation which presents a challenge to Western societies, in which 'white assumptions and white amnesia' (Cohen, 2017) have reigned for so long. We see this struggle expressed in debates about what should be memorialised, and which memorials should be removed or replaced. These same debates echo within the arts therapies where norms are being questioned and subaltern histories and perspectives are circulating with increasing frequency (see Dokter & Sajnani, 2023). In sites of teaching and practice, symbolic expression continues to facilitate attention to contradiction and paradox. However, as Savfi noted, attention to complexity and contradiction should not be confused with justice, which remains vital to healing. Condoling a death should not be confused with condoning, forgetting or enabling current manifestations of colonialism. Removing a statue should not be confused with the need to sustain efforts to disrupt the long-held beliefs and ideologies that memorials represent(ed) and provide reparations. The transgressive efforts of artists experimenting with how we experience cultural memory in the public sphere offer options for how we might call attention to the spaces between cultural extremes and the polarities of absence and presence.

Notes

1 Keynote address from ECArTE 2022 in Vilnius, see: https://bit.ly/ecartekeynote2022
2 News footage, see: https://bit.ly/queenspassing

References

Baldwin, J., Hughes, L., Hansberry, L., Capouya, E. & Kazin, A. (n.d.). The Negro in American Culture: A Group Discussion. [Video]. *YouTube*. Available at: https://www.youtube.com/watch?v=jNpitdJSXWY (Accessed January 3, 2024).

Cohen, R. (2017). Confederate statues and American memory. *The New York Times* (September 6, 2017). Retrieved from: https://www.nytimes.com/2017/09/06/opinion/confederate-statues-trump.html (Accessed January 3, 2024).

deWitte, M., Orkibi, H., Zarate, R., Karkou, V., Sajnani, N., Malhotra, B., Ho, R.T.H., Kaimal, G., Baker, F.A. & Koch, S.C. (2021). From therapeutic factors to mechanisms of change in the creative arts therapies: A scoping review. *Frontiers in Psychology*, July, 15(12), 678397. doi: 10.3389/fpsyg.2021.678397

Dickson, C. (2016). Dance under the swastika: Rudolf von Laban's influence on Nazi power. *International Journal of Undergraduate Research and Creative Activities*, 8(7). doi: http://dx.doi.org/10.7710/2168-0620.1063

Dokter, D. & Sajnani, N. (2023). *Intercultural dramatherapy: Imagination and action and the intersections of difference*. Oxford: Routledge.

Draaisma, D. (2000). *Metaphors of memory: A history of ideas about the mind*. Cambridge: Cambridge University Press.

Du Bois, W.E.B. (2008). *The souls of Black folk* (B.H. Edwards, Ed.). Oxford: Oxford University Press.

Eberhard-Kaechele, M. (2012). Memory, metaphor, and mirroring in movement therapy with trauma patients. In S. Koch, T. Fuchs, M. Summa & C. Muller (Eds.), *Body memory, metaphor, and movement* (pp. 267–287). Amsterdam: John Benjamins Publishing Company. https://doi.org/10.1075/aicr.84.21ebe

Fernandes, C. (2016). *The moving researcher: Laban/Bartenieff Movement Analysis in performing arts education and creative Arts therapies*. London: Jessica Kingsley.

Freud, S. (1930). *Civilization and its discontents*. London: Hogarth.

Hougham, R. & Jones, B. (2017). *Dramatherapy: Reflections and praxis*. London: Red Globe Press.

Leite, T. (2003). Music, metaphor and "Being with the Other": Music therapy with psychiatric patients. *Voices: A World Forum for Music Therapy*, *3*(2). Retrieved from: https://voices.no/index.php/voices/issue/view/273

Lisauskaitė, D. (2022). New de-Sovietisation law takes aim at Lithuania's remaining Soviet-era signs. *LRT*, June 6, 2022. Available at: https://www.lrt.lt/en/news-in-english/19/1711669/new-desovietisation-law-takes-aim-at-lithuania-s-remaining-soviet-era-signs (Accessed January 15, 2024).

Mann, S. (1996). Metaphor, symbol and the healing process in Dramatherapy. *Dramatherapy*, *18*(2), 2–5. https://doi.org/10.1080/02630672.1996.9689413

Moore, M. (2020, July 14). Absences and reminders: Searching for Soviet statues in the Baltics. *Deep Baltic*, July 14, 2020. Available at: https://deepbaltic.com/2020/07/14/absences-and-reminders-searching-for-soviet-statues-in-the-baltics/ (Accessed January 3, 2024).

Moon, B.L. (2007). *The role of metaphor in art therapy: Theory, method, and experience*. Springfield: Charles C. Thomas.

Nielsen, M.V. (2021, November 29). Moss fails to heal the wounds of Lithuania's memory wars. *New East Digital Archive*. Available at: https://www.new-east-archive.org/articles/show/13311/memory-wars-soviet-union-lithuania-petras-cvirka-monument-art-installation-moss-statue (Accessed January 3, 2024).

Ramsden, E. & Landy, R. (2021). Role theory and role method. In D.R. Johnson & R. Emunah (Eds), *Current Approaches in Drama Therapy*. 3rd edn. Springfield: Charles C. Thomas.

Roediger, H.L. (1980). Memory metaphors in cognitive psychology. *Memory and Cognition*, *8*(3), 231–246. https://doi.org/10.3758/bf03197611

Sapolsky, R. (2010). This is your brain on metaphors. *New York Times*, November 14, 2010. Available at: https://archive.nytimes.com/opinionator.blogs.nytimes.com/2010/11/14/this-is-your-brain-on-metaphors/ (Accessed January 3, 2024).

Smeijsters, H. (2012). Analogy and metaphor in music therapy. Theory and practice. *Nordic Journal of Music Therapy*, *21*(3), 227–249. https://doi.org/10.1080/08098131.2011.649299

Thibodeau, P.H. & Boroditsky, L. (2011). Metaphors we think with: The role of metaphor in reasoning. *PLOS ONE*, *6*(2), e16782. https://doi.org/10.1371/journal.pone.0016782

Törneke, N. (2010). *Learning RFT: An introduction to relational frame theory and its clinical applications*. Reno: Context Press.

Young, J. & Wood, L. (2018). Laban: A guide figure between dance/movement therapy and drama therapy. *Arts in Psychotherapy* 57, 11–19. http://dx.doi.org/10.1016/j.aip.2017.09.002

2

UNLOCKING MEMORY KNOTS

Encountering Self in the Multisensory Art Therapy Process

Audronė Brazauskaitė

Abstract

This article will theorise the process of the masterclass Unlocking Memory Knots, which was designed specifically for the 2022 ECArTE conference Memory, Shaping Connections in the Arts Therapies in Vilnius. In this hands-on experience, all participants were presented with different fabrics tied in knots or braids. They were asked to freely choose one braid and untie it to untangle the knot. Using the act of untying a knot they were asked to create free association and images that were revealed to them. Participants had different art mediums to create their freely associated images.

This process can be understood from several aspects: anthropological, psychoanalytical interpretation and sensory experience. What is the anthropological significance of weaving, knotting, braiding and untying in ancient cultures? We know that many mythologies explain the world as a cloth or web and that the universe is created by spinning or weaving. A knot is a cross, it is binding, fixing and at the same time locking, hiding a secret and protecting. The symbolic tying of the knot is inseparable from birth, death and wedding customs. Every mystery or riddle is a knot, and finding the answer is untying the knot. In Buddhism, there is a term "inner knots".

Psychotherapeutic action always aims to make the unconscious conscious. By touching and exploring braids made of different fabrics, participants become more open to subconscious images thanks to the sensory/tactile experience. Fabrics and other art materials, provoking different sensations, play an important role in the art therapy process, triggering associations and contributing to creative expression. The experience of the masterclass showed that most participants created images

DOI: 10.4324/9781032663944-2

about their primary relationship with their parents or other significant relationships. Of the ties of love, dependence, uncertainty and jealousy, the famous psychiatrist R.D. Laing (1970) said, "Words that come to mind to name them are: knots, tangles, fankles, impasses, disjunctions, "hirligigs, binds" (p. 7).

Based on the experience of the masterclass, this article will look at the connections between anthropological meaning, sensory experience and psychoanalytic interpretation and how these concepts intertwine in the creative process of art therapy.

Keywords: knot, weaving, plait, anthropological, art therapy, implicit memory, sensory, art materials, early memories, unconsciously, creative process

Abstract in Lithuanian

Santrauka

Atminties mazgų atrišimas: susitikimas su savimi multisensoriniame dailės terapijos procese

Šiame straipsnyje bus siekiama teoriškai pagrįsti meistriškumo klasės "Atminties mazgų atrišimas" procesą. Ši meistriškumo klasė buvo sukurta ir vyko 2022 m. Vilniuje ECArTE konferencijoje "Atmintis, formuojant ryšius meno terapijoje". Šios praktinės patirties metu visiems dalyviams buvo pristatytos kirting audinių surištos pynutės / mazgai. Jų buvo paprašyta laisvai pasirinkti vieną pynę ir atrišti, kad išsipainiotų mazgas. Atrišant mazgą, jų buvo paprašyta sukurti laisvą asociaciją ir atskleistus vaizdus. Dalyviai turėjo įvairių meno priemonių, kad galėtų kurti laisvai susietus vaizdinius.

Šis procesas gali būti pagrįstas tokiais aspektais: antropologine, psichologine ir jutimine patirtimi. Kokia antropologinė audimo, mezgimo, pynimo ir atrišimo reikšmė senovės kultūrose? Žinome, kad daugelis mitologijų pasaulį aiškina kaip audinį ar tinklą, kad visata sukurta verpimo ar pynimo būdu. Mazgas yra kryžius, jis riša, fiksuoja ir tuo pačiu užrakina, slepia paslaptį ir saugo. Simbolinis mazgo rišimas neatsiejamas nuo gimimo, mirties, vestuvių papročių. Kiekviena paslaptis ar mįslė yra mazgas, o atsakymo radimas reiškia mazgo išrišimą. Budizme yra terminas "vidiniai mazgai".

Psichoterapiniais veiksmais visada siekiama, kad nesąmoningas žmogus taptų labiau sąmoningu. Liesdami ir tyrinėdami pynes, pagamintas iš skirtingų audinių, dalyviai tampa atviresni pasąmonės vaizdiniams dėl jutiminės / lytėjimo patirties. Meistriškumo klasės patirtis parodė, kad visi dalyviai kūrė vaizdus apie savo pirminius santykius su tėvais ar kitus reikšmingus santykius. Garsus psichiatras R. D. Laingas vadina mazgais meilės, priklausomybės, netikrumo, pavydo ryšius: "Žodžiai, kurie ateina į galvą jiems pavadinti, yra mazgai, raizginiai, aklavietės, sūkuriai, surišimai".

Remiantis meistriškumo klasėje įgyta patirtimi, šiame straipsnyje bus nagrinėjamos sąsajos tarp antropologinės prasmės, juslinės patirties ir psichologinės interpretacijos bei kaip šios sąvokos susipina kūrybiniame dailės terapijos procese

> Humans are part of the fabric of all created matter.
>
> *Harold Searles (1960, p. 127)*

The title "Unlocking Memory Knots" encompasses a series of questions: what do the knots symbolise? how are they related to memory? why would one need to unlock them? The answers will be analysed through the following steps with the intention of expanding the understanding of knots: symbolic meaning and anthropological analysis, the tactile/sensory experience, the neuroscientific explanation, psychological and psychoanalytical interpretation and realisation through experience. From the early cultures, knots, plaiting, tying and weaving have occupied an important place in the rites of initiation, marriage, birth and death. A knot is an archetypal image, rooted in the human psyche, symbolising transformation, the passage into another state or stage of life. The art of weaving and textiles has played an important role throughout history, creating and maintaining social connections and communities (Celms, 2012; Tumėnas, 2011; Terry, 2020).

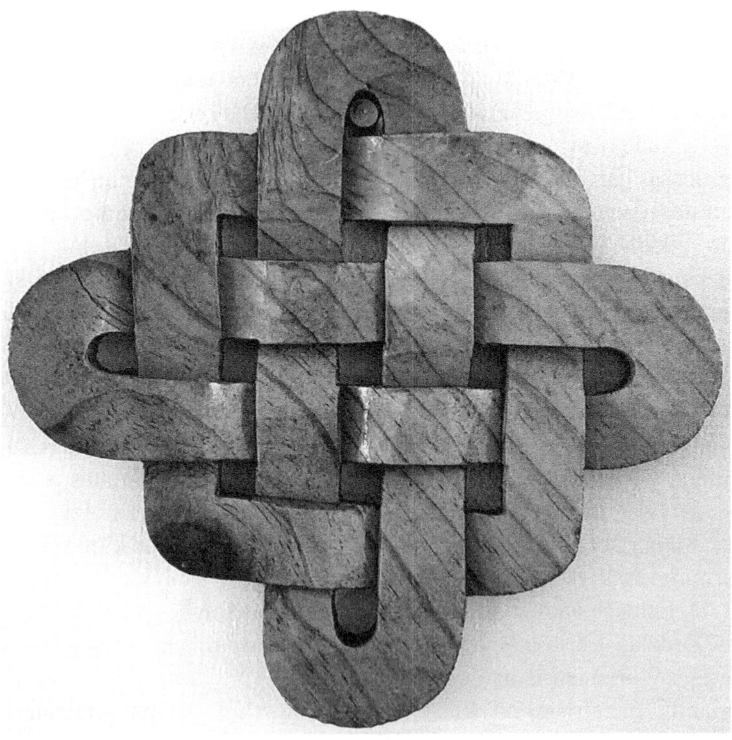

FIGURE 2.1 The Buddhist symbol: infinity knot. Photo credit: Audronė Brazauskaitė.

The metaphor "inner knots", which represents difficult unrecognised emotions and experiences, exists in Buddhist psychology and psychoanalysis. Untangling internal knots is acknowledging one's difficult experiences, looking at them with an accepting gaze. This leads to inner healing and recovery (Thich Nhat Hanh, 2019; Petric, 2022; Laing, 1970). This complex process of inner transformation is not easily understood, especially not when expressed verbally.

Therefore, the process of art therapy is especially suitable because the participants can give colours and shapes to their tangled experiences. Art therapy tools and materials such as paint, clay, paper, pencils and all the other materials, stimulate our visual, tactile, olfactory and auditory senses. Thanks to our implicit memory, this sensory stimulation evokes recollection through associations. Implicit memory also forms mental models, and unconscious processing affects behaviour, feelings and thoughts. We can recall a great deal of information through touch (Bonino *et al.*, 2008). Creating art products in art therapy has the effect of incorporating the whole psychosomatic cycle from sensations to early memories and gives shape and colour to one's autobiographic story. Hence art facilitates a continuous recreation and reinterpretation of memories. (Rubin, 2001; Hinz, 2009; Vance & Wahlin, 2008; Hass-Cohen & Carr, 2008).

A personal artistic practice allows for the art therapist to create original art therapy activities. For the author of this article, knots, plaiting, tying and weaving have been familiar and widely interpreted topics during her career as an

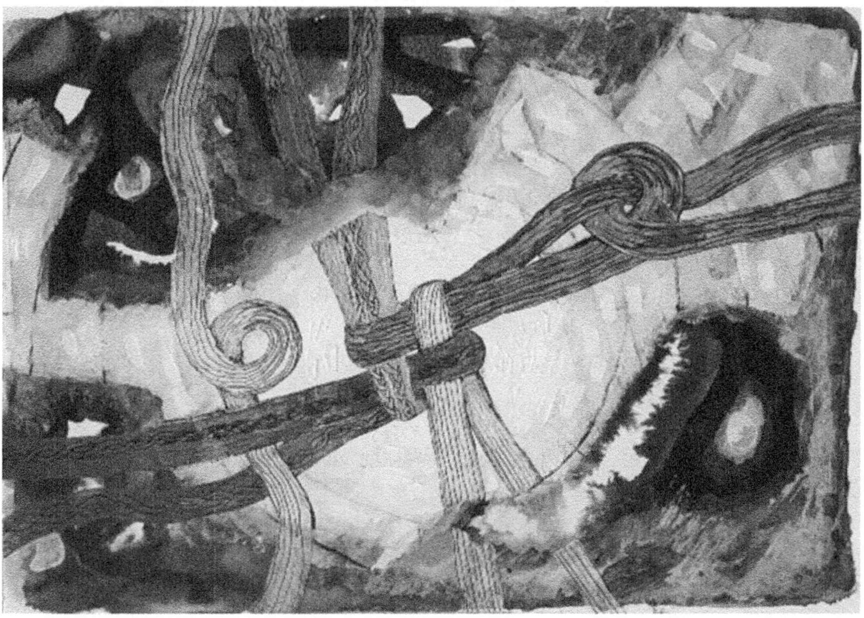

FIGURE 2.2 Author's drawing. Photo credit: Audronė Brazauskaitė.

artist/painter. One chanced upon this image of (un)tying knots spontaneously while drawing them and associating them intuitively with a specific period in the personal life during which one experienced separation from an important person. The author has been developing this knot imagery since then using different art media, to reflect what they meant to her. Using this as a foundation, an experiential art therapy task is developed. The goal is to grasp an affective memory through a spontaneous and associative process triggered by the untying of a knot. This idea is also closely based on an experience described by Sigmund Freud, where he would encourage his patients to visualise something, in order to recall forgotten memories:

> I placed my hands on the patient's forehead or took her head between my hands and said: "You will think of it under the pressure of my hands. At the moment at which I relax my pressure you will see something in front of you or something will come into your head. Catch hold of it. It will be what we are looking for – well, what have you seen or what has occurred to you?"
>
> *(Freud & Breuer, 1893–1895, p. 110)*

All the masterclass participants are presented with plaits or knots made of strips of fabric with various surfaces, which they can freely and spontaneously select. They are asked to choose one plait and untie, or untangle, the knot. Participants are instructed to be mindful of the action of untying, and once the knot is undone, to create a free association with it by drawing images. The emphasis on the metaphor of "unlocking one's knot" prompts the visualisation of an associated image, that participants can recreate using art tools and materials of their choice, from those provided. This allows them to freely create associated images. Interestingly, all participants create images about their early relationships with a parent, or other important primary relationships. Drawing from the experience of this masterclass, this article is going to consider the connections between the anthropological meaning, the sensory experience and its psychoanalytical interpretation, and investigate how these concepts intertwine in the creative art therapy process.

Untying as rites of passage: individual and community

From an anthropological standpoint, what do weaving, knotting, plaiting and (un)tying symbolise in ancient cultures? A variety of mythologies explain the world as a fabric or a net – the universe having been created by spinning or weaving. A knot is a cross, a bond, something anchored and, at the same time, locked, a secret, a kind of protection. Symbolic (un)tying is an intrinsic part of birth, death and marriage rites. Every secret or riddle is a knot and finding the

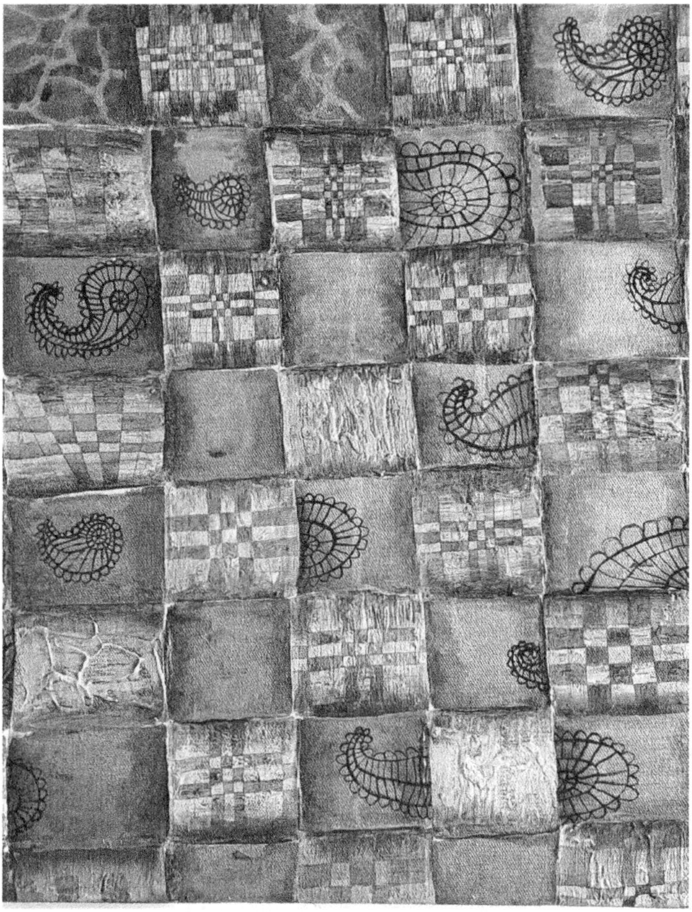

FIGURE 2.3 Author's drawing. Photo credit: Audronė Brazauskaitė.

answer parallels untying it. When we consider the action of tying and untying a knot from the anthropological viewpoint, we find some interesting explanations. Claude Lévi-Strauss (1997), an anthropologist and mythologist, discovered that the main themes that run through the rituals of early cultures are the creation of the world, setting various rules and schemes, defining blood and marital relationships, using crafts (weaving, pottery, smithery, construction and cooking), that are closely related to ceremonial acts. There are many studies which analyse the connection between weaving technologies as a semantic code, a sort of "technological gestalt", and the traditional ceremonial Indo-European poetry, folk narratives, mythologies and a holistic understanding of the world. Vytautas Tumėnas (2011) investigated the meaning and symbolism of fabrics and weaving in wedding customs, their mythological connection with the otherworld and the whole social, natural and spiritual cosmos, as well as life on earth and the human condition within the traditional Lithuanian worldview. Restyling the bride's hair in a special ceremony by undoing plaits and brushing the hair generally recreates the main moves of spinning and weaving. Twisting, plaiting and winding is a very common ceremonial metaphor. The main purpose of a piece of thread or rope is to use it to plait, weave, knit or knot. These actions give birth to a piece of fabric or expand it in space. According to Vladimir Toporov (2000), the mythopoetic metaphors of textile artefacts semantically play with the following properties: extension, the ability to join separate and often polar objects on the one hand, or rupturing, the loss of ability, having an end(ing) on the other hand. This range of properties directly relates to the most prominent thread metaphors, those of life, destiny, time, path, sacrifice and binding, as a synonym of contact. In ceremonies, a piece of thread or a sash symbolises the integration of the hero into the social structure. Mircea Eliade (1980), who investigated the symbolism of the archetype of ropes, loops, knots, and tangles in the mythologies of Indo-European and neighbouring peoples and indeed the rituals and beliefs of different nations around the world, concluded that in mythical characters, this archetype is associated with magical powers, the ability to both kill and bring back from the dead, to harm and heal. In ceremonial practice, the archetype of tying shows up as a magical or religious power, a symbol of initiation, important in all religions. Eliade also revealed the cosmological symbolism in Indian and Chinese mythologies of fabric and ties as representative of cosmic order and the universal bond. Dainius Razauskas (2000) also offers important insights into the etymological connections found in Indo-European languages between textile methodologies (tying, knitting, knotting, crocheting, spinning, weaving, winding, plaiting, binding), and textile artefacts (threads, ropes) on the one hand, and the images of streams, running water, rivers, swimming and ceremonial bathing on the other. According to Razauskas, untying has the characteristic of freeing or letting go as we witness in the flow of water away from its source.

As noted by Valdis Celms (2012), patterns are our (i.e., Balts:[1] Lithuanian, Latvian) thoughts about the world, as expressed in Balts ethnos. In the Lithuanian language, the word "raštas" is used to refer to the pattern of a piece of fabric and also the script – the text spelt out in letters and symbols in a book. This confirms the notion that these mental and physical processes are intimately related.

Weaving, knitting and textiles have always been an important cultural and social activity. A good example can be found in 20th-century Indian culture, when Mahatma Gandhi elevated the craft of spinning from an ethnographic activity of the rural economy to an element of the modern economy, a symbol of political ideology, national revival, unification and identity and, finally, to the spiritual, aesthetic and social education methods, attributing a spiritual meaning to it. Gandhi adopted the spinning technology that was popular in the Indian household and developed into an economic, cultural and ideological anticolonial movement of India, which helped to unify the society and shape the modern nation of India (Tumėnas, 2011).

Contemporary anthropologist Cristian Terry (2020) researched the role of textiles in the Andes. She proved that Andean textiles play many roles in Peru and Bolivia of both local and touristic significance (e.g., utilitarian, decorative, ceremonial, sentimental, identity-related, economic and so on). Adopting the Actor Network Theory approach to social theory, the researcher perceives Andean textiles as an important non-human actor, constantly interacting with people. For example, it features in shaman rituals, when ponchos are used as a local identity performance and when material souvenirs are purchased to remind one of the travel experiences. Andean textiles inspire social change among rural and urban dwellers – weavers, artists, designers and retailers. In addition to the social change from weaving, the weaving practice itself is changing too. In other words, a new fashionable, industrial and hybrid production has been developed which caters more for the urban and/or tourist market, which, in turn, provides money for social change. Hence, it seems that these two ideas are interlaced and closely related to the market: social change and changes in weaving methodology intertwine in the contemporary reality of the Andes.

Hence, right from the early cultures, knots, plaiting, tying and weaving have occupied an important place in the rites of initiation, marriage, birth and death. A knot is an archetypal image, rooted in the human psyche, symbolising transformation, the passage into another state or stage of life. The art of weaving and textiles have played an important role throughout history, creating and maintaining social connections and articulating community values.

Encountering oneself

In the masterclass Unlocking Memory Knots, the metaphor of unlocking the knots is a central idea that all participants explore through visual creation. Participants enact and embody this metaphor and then draw what awakens in them as individual meanings. In Buddhist psychology, there is the term "inner knots" – these are certain sensory experiences that, depending on one's reactions, seem to tie knots in us. When it is difficult for an individual to admit their anger, fear or disappointment, they use strong defence mechanisms that deny the existence of these feelings – this is how internal knots are created. Buddhist monk and teacher Thich Nhat Hanh says, in order to protect each other's happiness, we must be aware of and report our inner knots as soon as they arise, talk about them and untangle them. Discovering inner knots, interacting with them and making new connections is a path of self-knowledge that continues in creativity. Donima Petric (2022) says that mental knots consist of negative emotions, feelings (subconscious knots) and tangled thoughts that are not purposeful but pathological and disabling. Psychic knots have many harmful consequences for both emotional and cognitive life. The goal of knot psychotherapy is to untangle these knots. In his book *Knots*, Scottish psychoanalyst. Laing (1970) describes different relationship and behaviour patterns and scenarios that are formed in early childhood in the form of poems and dialogues. Laing's extremely simple minimalist text is painfully candid about the types of attachments and their dynamics in the psyche, in terms of patterns of behaviours which repeat themselves in different situations. He describes different relations – love bonds, dependence, deception, jealousy between lovers, between parents and children, between analysts and patients or all of these together – as knots: "Words that come to mind to naming them are: knots, tangles, fankles, impasses, disjunctions, Whirligigs, binds" (p. 7).

MY MOTHER LOVES ME.
I FEEL GOOD.
I FEEL GOOD BECAUSE SHE LOVES ME.
I AM GOOD BECAUSE I FEEL GOOD.
I FEEL GOOD BECAUSE I AM GOOD.
MY MOTHER LOVES ME BECAUSE I AM GOOD.
MY MOTHER DOES NOT LOVE ME.
I FEEL BAD.
I FEEL BAD BECAUSE SHE DOES NOT LOVE ME.
I AM BAD BECAUSE I FEEL BAD.
I FEEL BAD BECAUSE I AM BAD.
I AM BAD BECAUSE SHE DOES NOT LOVE ME.
SHE DOES NOT LOVE ME BECAUSE I AM BAD.

Very often, our knotted states are simply difficult to understand. The essence of art therapy and the ability to visually represent what is difficult to put into words is a great way to acknowledge and untie internal knots. By giving colour and shape to your knots, it becomes easier to untie them, see them and understand them. Such a process is accompanied by strong insights. Judy Rubin (2001) says:

> I find the use of art in an uncovering, insight-oriented approach to be the most powerful and exciting kind of art therapy for myself, as well as for most of my patients. The shock of discovering previously unknown and usually unwanted aspects of self is often visceral. The excitement of not only seeing,

> but also feeling connections between what has been known and what has been hidden is equally powerful. Insight in good analytic art therapy is no intellectual matter; it is a vivid awareness, which allows all kinds of things that once seemed inexplicable to make sense. When they are deeply felt, grasped, and accepted, the internal shifts which lead to genuine and lasting change can be truly amazing.
>
> *(p. 18).*

The metaphor of inner knots, which represents difficult unrecognised emotions and experiences, exists in Buddhist psychology and psychoanalysis (Hanh, 2019; Petric, 2022; Laing, 1970). Untangling internal knots is acknowledging one's difficult experiences and looking at them with an accepting gaze. This leads to inner healing and recovery. This complex process of inner transformation is not easily understood, especially not when expressed verbally. Therefore, the process of art therapy facilitates in the individual a personalised method by which they are able to confront the moment of entanglement and give it a definite visual representation.

Tactility and neuroscience

Art therapy is medium-specific and relies upon the particular art tool and material that is being employed (e.g., paint, clay, pencils, felt tips, different kinds of paper, etc.). Each of these materials has different physical forms and, with that, a potential for provoking different sensations. All these materials play an important part in the art therapy process, triggering associations and contributing to the language of creative expression. Sensory stimulation through music, movement and painting can often develop memory functions, claims Liza Hinz (2009). Knots and plaits used in the masterclass are made of different textiles and produce different tactile sensations. Participant testimonies show that it is this aspect of touching different textile surfaces that evokes strong associations for many, and unexpectedly, taking them back to early memories. Hence this paper would further analyse the ways art therapy stimulates memory processes, as well as the mechanics of how the tactile experience inspires associations and memories.

Paint, clay, paper, pencils and other materials used in art therapy stimulate our vision, hearing and senses of touch and smell. Participants see various bright or muted colours, different shapes and lines and their combinations. Participants touch, stroke and squeeze surfaces that are slimy, damp, wet, cold, warm, sharp and soft. They smell clay, paint and all the other items they are asked to use. They hear sounds that different materials make while being manipulated in the creative process. This multisensory creative experience triggers associations and related memories. Without their noticing, the sensorial abundance in the art therapy process suddenly takes them to an unconscious level where specific associations and memories reside. Researchers claim that the memories which affect us unconsciously thanks to our earlier experience are stored in our implicit memory. Robin Vance and Kara Wahlin (2008) say that implicit memories refer to somatic/bodily perceptual experiences, which include memories of how things looked or smelled as well as our emotions and moods at the time. Implicit memory starts to form in infancy even before the age of nine months. It's one of the two main types of long-term human memory that doesn't require conscious awareness. It directs actions, reactions, and body responses with little or no conscious effort, involving multiple brain structures. The amygdala, hippocampus and medial prefrontal cortex support fear conditioning and emotional memory, the basal ganglia and motor cortex support behavioural memory, the parietal and occipital cortices facilitate perceptual memory, and the parietal cortex stores bodily memories (Carlson, in Vance & Wahlin, 2008). Implicit memory builds up unconscious generalised summaries of experiences, which help us learn from the past, anticipate future experiences and quickly react to survival threats. Siegel (1999) remarks that implicit memory primes us for survival from threats of all kinds (suggesting that implicit memory forms mental models, unconscious processing and influences behaviours, feelings and thoughtsVance and Wahlin notice that sometimes we may believe our decisions are based on our objective review of available data and possible choices, but mostly our decisions about who we are and what we do are based upon the bubbling up of quick implicit memories, sensations and projections. By our first birthday, many patterns of implicit memory are firmly built into the brain. Repeated attachment experiences, positive or negative, are juggled in the neural networks of the brain, so much so that they become personality traits of the person. This juggling happens automatically – outside of recall – and informs who we are and who we will become. Sensations and projections evoke memories, but, on the other hand, our emotional state resonates with certain external triggers. Robin Vance and Kara Wahlin summarise that emotion and memory are capable of exerting powerful influences on the processing of sensory material. For example, physically and emotionally abused children have difficulty taking their attention away from an angry face. Emotions also bias attention to the perception of mood-congruent stimuli. Emotional situations create especially vivid, long-lasting memories, known as flashbulb memories. These can form as a response to a unique public event that intensely affects millions of people (Vance & Wahlin, 2008).

Masterclass participants who took part in the art therapy session highlighted that strong memories were particularly rekindled by touching the materials. Therefore, this paper touches upon the research that addresses the information we acquire through our sense of touch. Researchers Bonino *et al.* (2008)

emphasise that the brain's response to a tactile memory task is not solely related to visual images and that people born blind can successfully interact with their surroundings through touch.

Researchers Stadtlander *et al.* (1998) investigated how different age groups recall information when presented in different ways (visual-only, visual-and-haptic, haptic-only). The data showed that younger adults remembered more than older adults under all conditions. However, both age groups had the highest recall under the haptic conditions.

In making art products, participants activate many procedural and autobiographical choices while forming a visual narrative. Therapeutic encouragement reinforces their sense of agency, and art-making allows the participants to adjust past views/beliefs about their abilities to express themselves. Successful art-making enhances the memory of the self as capable. Vivid visual images activate working memory and augment the older, previously stored information. Therefore, the recall of events, especially if they are emotionally charged, is often drastically different from what actually happened. We keep on updating the altered memories (LeDoux, in Vance & Wahlin, 2008). Art pieces are memories in constant re-creation.

So, art therapy tools and materials such as paint, clay, paper, pencils and all the other materials, stimulate our visual, tactile, olfactory and auditory senses. Thanks to our implicit memory, this sensory stimulation evokes associations and memories. Implicit memory also forms mental models, and unconscious processing affects behaviour, feelings and thoughts. We can recall a great deal of information through touch. Through creating art products in art therapy, we incorporate the whole psychosomatic cycle from sensations to early memories and give shape and colour to our autobiographic story. In art, memories are constantly being re-created and reinterpreted.

Experiential cases

This section presents the participants' feedback on the felt experiences of the Unlocking Memory Knots masterclass. All information and drawings are shared with the permission of the participants. The names of the participants have been changed and their identities have not been revealed. Interestingly, many of the art therapy masterclass participants' images and reflections expressed their early memories with their primary caregivers (mother and father). It is important to note that the early memories came from touching the knots/braids with their fingers. Participants touched, stroked, and rummaged through materials and sensations, and then these sensations created memories. As Robin Vance and Kara Wahlin (2008) argue, implicit memories refer to somatic/bodily perceptual experiences, including memories of how things looked or smelled as well as our emotions and moods at the time.

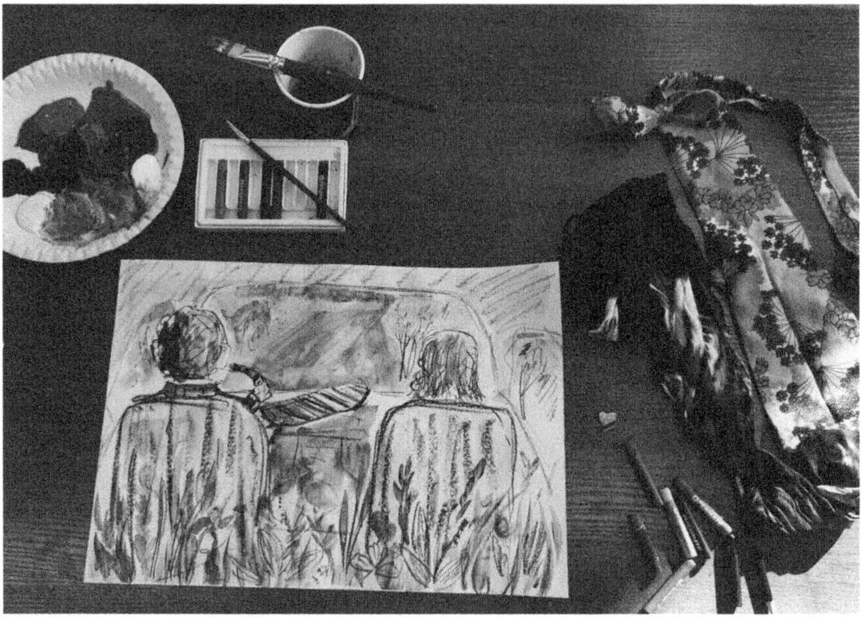

FIGURE 2.4 Participant's drawing: Laura. Photo credit: Audronė Brazauskaitė.

Participant Laura

After receiving the instructions, I chose one knot that I liked the most. A man's tie was tied between two pieces of cloth. It was relevant to me as a costume designer. Touching the different textures of the fabric with my fingers, I explored them and admired the blending of colours. My thoughts returned me to my childhood. I remembered my dad because ties of this style were fashionable in his youth. I remembered my father's striped tie, his brown suit, I could feel the texture of the fabric – it was so deeply etched in my memory. I was sitting in the back seat of the family car, and I could see the backs of my father and mother in the front. And that smell of the first smoke of a freshly lit cigarette (around 1980, it was still quite normal to smoke in the car and elsewhere). . . I will remember it all my life. . . The memories followed each other causing strong nostalgic feelings.

Participant Mary

At the masterclass-workshop called Unlocking Memory Knots – I felt untangled. Literally and figuratively, the material shreds were untied and which in turn also untangled memories starting from infancy, vividly touching on the importance of female relatives (i.e., mother and grandmothers) in my life, ending with the present. It was one of the two materials that I found particularly pleasant to touch and that had to do with the gauze I used to sleep with when I was a baby. During the drawing process, I unconsciously wrapped it around my palm. The whole time while I was drawing like this, I felt a pleasant warmth, and only towards the end of the process did I realise what a significant meaning I gave to the piece of material; both through my body (palms) and in the drawing (the need for care, embrace, security). Untying the knot itself did not cause discomfort, but it gave me enough time to feel the quality of the material. So, in my case, the most important thing here was the materiality – one piece of material was cotton, which was the reason for my inner journey through time, and the other piece, which was different in texture, composition and colour, I did not like and after untangling it I put it aside without any doubt, that way focusing all of my attention on the cotton and immersing myself in memories and associations surrounding them.

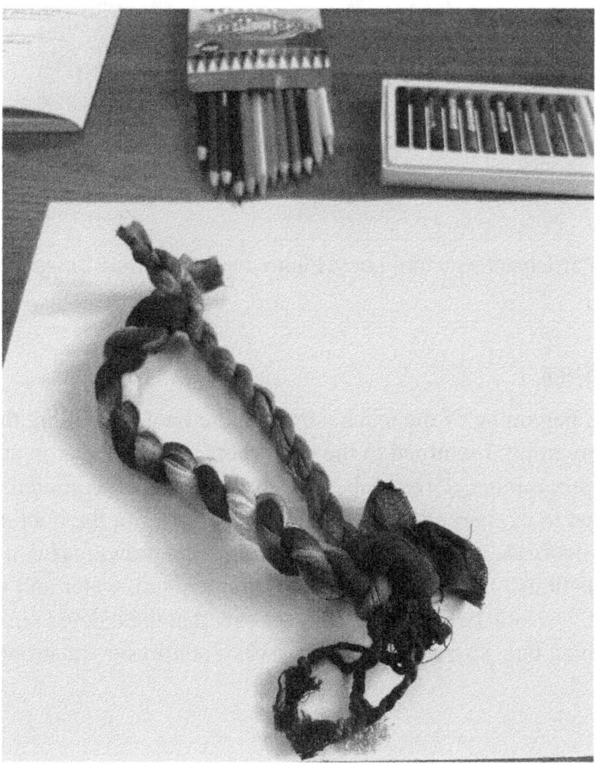

FIGURE 2.5 Participant's drawing: Mary. Photo credit: Audronė Brazauskaitė.

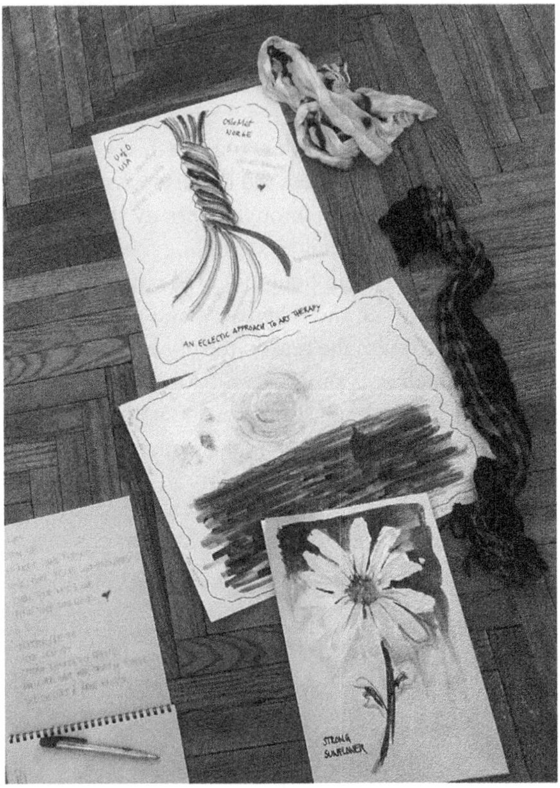

FIGURE 2.6 Participant's picture Lucy. Photo credit: Audronė Brazauskaitė.

Participant Lucy

I liked the beginning of the touch, stroking the knot and letting the memories come to my mind. I returned to the US, where I spent a year in an art therapy master's programme. I remembered drawing a multi-coloured braid when I was asked to explain my approach to art therapy. So, the knot in this workshop sent me back 30 years! When we did the first drawing (I don't remember the "instructions") I made an image of summer, sun, water and wrote words like peace, warmth, belonging, family – I saw that the colours reminded me of the Ukrainian flag, so my next drawing was a sunflower – a strong sunflower.

Participant Barbara

After receiving the assignment and taking the braided braid from the ribbons, I studied the colours. Then I braided it a little, separated it. After that, more

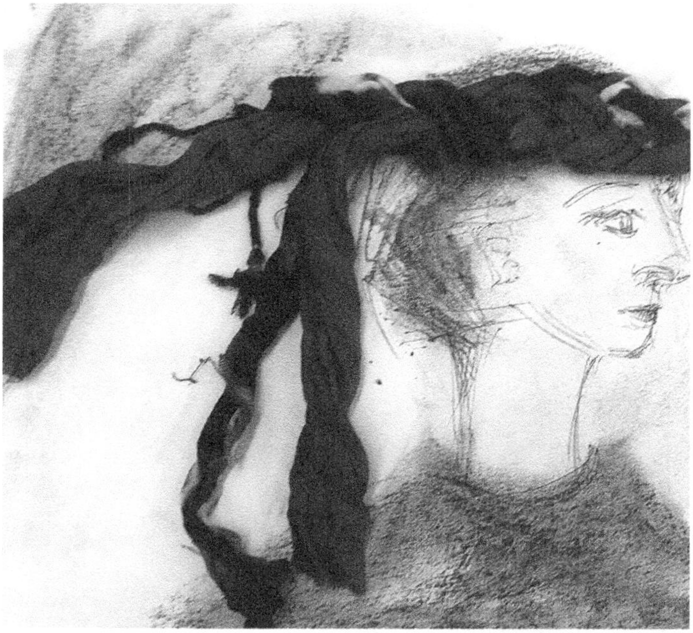

FIGURE 2.7 Participant's drawing: Barbara. Photo credit: Audronė Brazauskaitė.

and more. The hidden colours opened up. I enjoyed. Then I stretched it out on the table, wrapped it on my hand, rolled . . . Later I started braiding the ribbons like a braid. Brought to childhood about the braided bun about the cut hair . . . I was ten years old. My hair used to be thick, my mother kept washing it with vinegar to make it shiny. Everyone raved about how beautiful the thick braided hair was. When combing, my hair pulled and it hurt, so we got into a fight with my mother. I don't know how it was there, whether I wanted it myself or my mother, but they cut my hair. It was very strange. The weight of the head disappeared; it became easy. I received many compliments. But it was a strange feeling. Who am I, a girl or a boy? I missed that hair braid. At the same time, my maturity was delayed. I drew a picture, a face like a child, like a girl, like a boy. Who am I? I drew with pastel and pen. The figure's clothes are blue. Lots of blue punctuating the pink, green and yellow in the drawing. Later, I added a braid woven from strips of fabric to the head of the drawn person. That's how I became a girl in the drawing. There came an understanding of that transformation, that important moment when you become a girl. What then happens in the body, sexuality, later pregnancy, etc. The last step I did was to make a headpiece like a crown out of ribbons of fabric braid and put it on top of the drawn woman. The image of a woman from the grandmother and older times, which in Lithuania was the

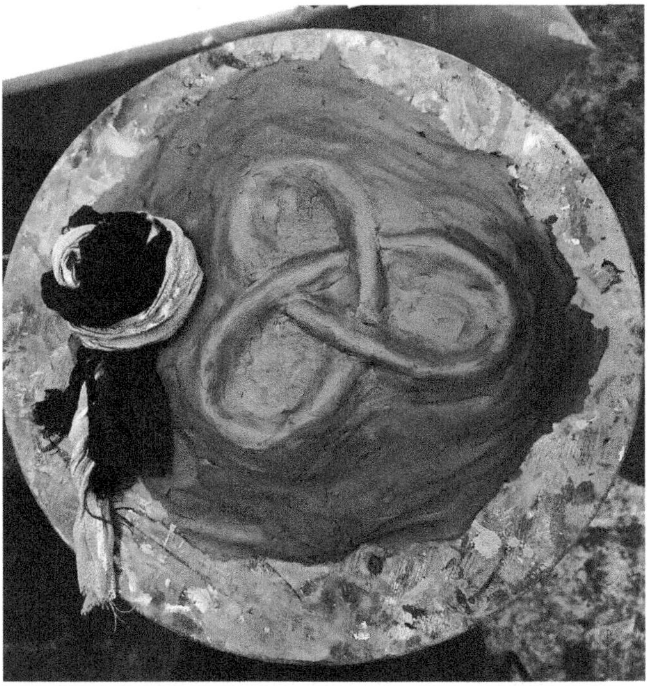

FIGURE 2.8 Participant's clay work: Helen. Photo credit: Audronė Brazauskaitė.

> image of a mature married woman. Both then and now, there was peace and self-acceptance from the point of maturity. Now the next time has come, the reproductive period ends. Courage to change, changing shapes, constructions in the drawing allowed to discover, see possibilities, resources in a new form, accept, express. The art therapy process in this workshop helped me to see the three stages of my life – little girl, young girl and matured woman; to feel the three transformations – to feel the possibilities of each stage. As of today, I am 55 years old. At this stage I am like in the ocean where I discover new stages of my age and forms of my being and forms in which it is good to be.

Some participants emphasised that the knot symbol, which has archetypal meaning in different cultures, helped to generalise and reinforce insights.

Participant Helen

> This was the connection to my heart and my soul. . . In this work I felt a healing process and regained trust. . . Which knots are created by myself – which

> do I carry as a heritage of my ancestors? Knots can be solved but they also support me. . . . I enjoyed the workshop very much. It brought my attention to my inner knots but in a friendly way. To accept that they also supported me, but that there is a time to undo them.

Participant Anne

> The created image helped me feel who I am, what is mine, and what other people's energy, emotions, feelings, and thoughts are. I named this drawing "Separateness, freedom".

As Liza D. Hinz (2009) underlines, symbols function as tools for finding solutions to problems on a higher level of integration.

Conclusion

After summarising the material presented in the article, we can see that, anthropologically, knots, braiding, tying and weaving have played an important role in the rituals of life creation/termination, marriages and initiation rituals since the earliest human cultures. The knot is an archetypal image rooted in people's consciousness and subconsciousness, signifying transformation and transition to another state or stage of life. In the course of history as well as in contemporary life, the art of weaving and textiles plays an important role in the creation and maintenance of social relations and communities. It's like creating a network or fabric of interpersonal relationships, thoughts, their synchronicity, contradictions and reflections. As discussed in the section Encountering Oneself, the metaphor of inner knots lives on in Buddhist psychology and psychoanalysis, in which it represents unacknowledged difficult emotions and experiences. Untangling internal knots is acknowledging one's difficult experiences and looking at them with an accepting gaze. This leads to inner healing and recovery. This complex process of inner transformation is facilitated through the processes of art. In the creative process of art an artist intimately, naturally and intuitively can reach these essential meanings of knotting/weaving action. Art therapy puts the participants in touch with their fragile affective moments that will otherwise slip through the recesses of their minds. The sensory stimulations of art therapy arise and make accessible certain critically untangled experiences of the self that are suddenly opened for reflection and examination. Like flowing streams, the participants witness a flow of emotional memories which they had held onto forever. The moment of letting go creates a lightness, in some cases, while feeling calmness in the act of returning to one's source.

In art therapy using paints, clay, paper, pencils and other materials affects visual, tactile, olfactory and aural sensations. Thanks to our involuntary memory, these sensory stimulations give rise to associations and memories. Because of this, the art therapy participant is exposed to the entire psychosomatic cycle – from sensations to early memories. They give colour and form to their autobiographical story. In works of art, memories are constantly re-created and re-perceived. The participants of the masterclass were presented with tied braids/knots made of textile materials which they could choose freely and spontaneously. They were asked to choose one braid and untie the knot. It is encouraged to be in the process and experience the act of untying the knot. The metaphor of untying the knot accompanied the participants towards visual creation – all participants drew, depicting their association. The experience of the masterclass demonstrated that participants mostly created images of their early relationship with their mother/father or other significant primary relationships. The rich process of art therapy – from a metaphorical action and different sensations, to representing and naming a symbol – allowed the participants of the masterclass to untie their inner knots and see themselves differently.

Acknowledgment

I sincerely thank the participants of the masterclass who shared their experience. Without you this article would not exist. I thank my daughter, Sibile, and my husband, Sudipto, for their support.

Note

1 The Balts or Baltic peoples (Lithuanian: baltai, Latvian: balti) are an ethno-linguistic group of peoples who speak the Baltic languages: Lithuanian, Latvian.

References

Bonino, D., Ricciardi, E., Sani, L., Gentili, C., Vanello, N., Guazzelli, M., Vecchi, T. and Pietrini, P. (2008). Tactile spatial working memory activates the dorsal extrastriate cortical pathway in congenitally blind individuals. *Archives Italiennes de Biologie, 146*(3–4): 133–146. https://europepmc.org/article/MED/19378878

Celms, V. (2012). *Baltų raštai ir ženklai: baltų pasaulio modelis, struktūra, vaizdiniai, simboliai.* Vilnius: Mintis.

Kandel, E.R. (2006). *In search of memory: The emergence of a new science of mind.* New York: W.W. Norton & Company.

Eliade, M. (1980). *Images et symbolcs. Esais sur le symbolismc magino-rcligieiix.* Paris: Editions Gallimard.

Eliade, M. (2011). *Obrazy i symbole.Szkice o symbolizmie magiczno-religijnym.* (Przelożyli: M. i P. Rodakowie). Warszawa: Wydawnict in Vytautas Tumėnas (2011) *Audimo technologijų erotinė ir iniciacinė reikšmė lietuvių kultūroje: simbolių choreografiniai ir naratyviniai atitikmenys komparatyvistiniu požiūriu in Antanas Andrijauskas* (ed.) Rytai-vakarai: komparatyvistinės studijos XI. Kultūrų sąveika.

Freud, S. and Breuer, J. 1893–1895, in J. Rubin (ed.). (2001). *Approaches to Art Therapy: theory and technique*, 2nd edn. New York: Routledge.

Hinz, L.D. (2009). *Expressive therapies continuum: A framework for using art in therapy*. New York: Routledge.

Munakata, Y., Casey, B.J. and Diamond, A. (2004) Developmental cognitive neuroscience: progress and potential. *Trends in Cognitive Sciences*, *8*(3), 2004, 122–128. https://doi.org/10.1016/j.tics.2004.01.005.

Laing, R.D. (1970). *Knots*. New York: Vintage, Random House.

LeDoux, J.E. (2000). Emotion circuits in the brain. *Annual Review of Neuroscience*, *23*, 155–184. https://doi.org/10.1146/annurev.neuro.23.1.155

Lévi-Strauss, C. (1997). *Laukinis mąstymas*. Vilnius: Baltos lankos, in Vytautas Tumėnas (2011) *Audimo technologijų erotinė ir iniciacinė reikšmė lietuvių kultūroje: simbolių choreografiniai ir naratyviniai atitikmenys komparatyvistiniu požiūriu in Antanas Andrijauskas* (ed.) Rytai-vakarai: komparatyvistinės studijos XI. Kultūrų sąveika.

Petric, D. (2022). The Knot Theory of Mind. *Open Journal of Medical Psychology*, *11*(1). doi: 10.13140/RG.2.2.27630.72009

Pillemer, D.B. (1998). *Momentous events, vivid memories*. Cambridge, MA: Harvard University Press.

Razauskas, D. (2000). *Ryto ratų ritimai*. Vilnius: Pradai, 174–181, in Vytautas Tumėnas (2011) *Audimo technologijų erotinė ir iniciacinė reikšmė lietuvių kultūroje: simbolių choreografiniai ir naratyviniai atitikmenys komparatyvistiniu požiūriu in Antanas Andrijauskas* (ed.) Rytai-vakarai: komparatyvistinės studijos XI. Kultūrų sąveika.

Rubin, J. (2001). Discovery, insight, and art therapy. In J.A. Rubin (ed.), *Approaches to art therapy: Theory and technique*, 2nd edn. New York: Routledge.

Searles, H. (1960). The nonhuman environment. In M. Hills de Zarate (2017), *Daiktai: materialioji kultūra ir tapatybės konstravimas (etnografinė perspektyva)* in Stanislovas Mostauskis, Audronė Brazauskaitė (ed.) *Menas terapija sveikata*, Kaunas: VDA Kauno fakultetas.

Siegel, D.J. (1999). *The developing mind: Towards a neurobiology of interpersonal experience*. New York and London: The Guilford Press.

Stadtlander L.M., Murdoch, L.D. and Heiser, S.M. (1998). Visual and haptic influences on memory: Age differences in recall. *Experimental Aging Research*, 24(3): 257–272. doi: 10.1080/036107398244247.

Terry, C. (2020). Weaving social change(s) or changes of weaving? The ethnographic study of Andean textiles in Cusco and Bolivia. *Artl@s Bulletin*, *9*(1), Article 6.

T.N. Hanh (2019). *How to fight*. New Delhi: Aleph Book Company.

Toporov. V. (2000). *Baltų mitologijos ir ritualo tyrimai*. Vilnius: Aidai.

Tumėnas. V. (2011). *Audimo technologijų erotinė ir iniciacinė reikšmė lietuvių kultūroje: simbolių choreografiniai ir naratyviniai atitikmenys komparatyvistiniu požiūriu* in Antanas Andrijauskas (ed.) Rytai-vakarai: komparatyvistinės studijos XI. Kultūrų sąveika.

Vance, R. and Wahlin, K. (2008). Memory and art. In N. Hass-Cohen and R. Carr (eds.), *Art therapy and clinical neuroscience*. London and Philadelphia: Jessica Kingsley Publishers.

van der Kolk, B.A. (1996). The complexity of adaptation to trauma: Self-regulation, stimulus discrimination, and characterological development. In B.A. van der Kolk, A.C. McFarlane and L. Weisaeth (eds.), *Traumatic stress: The effects of overwhelming experience on mind, body, and society*. New York: The Guilford Press.

Vöhringer, I.A., Kolling, T., Graf, F., Poloczek, S., Fassbender, I., Freitag, C., Lamm, B., Suhrke, J., Teiser, J., Teubert, T., Keller, H., Lohaus, A., Schwarzer, G. and Knopf, M. (2017). The development of implicit memory from infancy to childhood: On average performance levels and interindividual differences. *Child Development*, *89*(2): 370–382. doi: 10.1111/cdev.12749. https://pubmed.ncbi.nlm.nih.gov/28220933/

3

NEVER PAST

Embodied Memory in Humans and Other Animals

Gabriele Schmid

Abstract

"The past is never dead. It's not even past," William Faulkner famously wrote in *Requiem for a Nun*. The persistence of embodied memory is both a crucial moment of trauma and trauma therapy, and in the development of artistic works.

Today, the traumas of circulating viruses, extreme drought and severe conflicts have become part of our daily lives. We have embodied them. Embodied memory and the capacity of animals to share states of fear and other emotions are relevant in the artworks under discussion in this paper: works by the Belgian artist Berlinde De Bruyckere, the American artist Matthew Barney, the Lithuanian artist Eglė Budvytytė and the Ukrainian artist and co-founder of Femen, Oksana Shachko. Also, the interrelation of the human and non-human world plays a significant role in the four positions of these artists. Trauma is never far away though.

The different kinds of memories range from the cellular memory of the microbes in and around us to biographical and culturally embedded memories. Myth and religion play a significant role, whether explicit or implicit, embodied in the artist and their work.

According to the understanding of artistic research by Finnish researcher Juha Varto, the manifests of artists can be seen as part of their research and body of work. So, the artist's statements will be linked to concepts from scientific or literary fields, understood as analogies. According to the methodology of artistic (auto)ethnography, these fields are the contexts of artistic awareness and the developing artworks.

DOI: 10.4324/9781032663944-3

The potential of the artwork to act as a carrier of the present past (Faulkner) sheds light on the role that artistic creation may play in an artistic-therapeutic practice that deals with the struggle with a past that prevents us from achieving homeostasis and thus resilience.

Keywords: embodied memory, symbiosis, artistic research, post-humanism, trauma

Abstract in German

"Das Vergangene ist nicht tot; es ist nicht einmal vergangen", schrieb William Faulkner in "Requiem für eine Nonne". Das Fortbestehen des Körpergedächtnisses ist ein entscheidendes Moment in der Traumatherapie und zugleich bei der Entwicklung künstlerischer Werke.

Heute sind die Traumata von zirkulierenden Viren, extremer Trockenheit und schweren Konflikten Teil unseres täglichen Lebens geworden. Wir haben sie verinnerlicht. Das verkörperte Gedächtnis und die Fähigkeit von Tieren, Angstzustände und andere Emotionen mitzuteilen, sind in den Kunstwerken, die zur Sprache kommen, von Bedeutung. Auch die Wechselbeziehung zwischen der menschlichen und der nichtmenschlichen Welt spielt in den vier künstlerischen Positionen eine wichtige Rolle, wobei die Thematik des Traumas nie weit entfernt ist. Zur Sprache kommen die Arbeiten der belgischen Künstlerin Berlinde De Bruyckere und des amerikanischen Künstlers Matthew Barney, der litauischen Künstlerin Eglė Budvytytė und der ukrainischen Künstlerin und Mitbegründerin von Femen, Oksana Shachko.

Die verschiedenen Weisen von Erinnerungen reichen vom Zellgedächtnis der Mikroben in und um uns bis hin zu biografischen und kulturell verankerten Erinnerungen. Mythos und Religion spielen eine wichtige Rolle, ob explizit oder implizit, sozusagen verkörpert in den Künstler:innen und ihren Werken.

Nach Juha Vartos Verständnis von künstlerischer Forschung können die Manifeste von Künstler:innen als Teil ihrer Forschung und ihres Werks betrachtet werden. Im Text werden die Künstler:innenstatements mit wissenschaftlichen oder literarischen Konzepten verbunden, welche als Analogien verstanden werden. Gemäß der Methodik der künstlerischen (Auto-)Ethnographie sind diese Felder die Kontexte des künstlerischen Selbstverständnisses und der entstehenden Kunstwerke.

Das Potenzial von Kunstwerken, als Träger der gegenwärtigen Vergangenheit (Faulkner) zu fungieren, wirft ein Licht auf die Rolle, die künstlerisches Schaffen in einer künstlerisch-therapeutischen Praxis spielen kann, welche sich mit Erinnerungen befasst, die uns daran hindern, Homöostase und damit Resilienz zu erreichen.

"The past is never dead. It's not even past," William Faulkner (1951) famously wrote in *Requiem for a Nun*. The persistence of embodied memory is both a crucial moment of trauma and trauma therapy and in the development of artistic works. In common language, the use of the term 'trauma' does not only imply the traumatic event but also the aftermath. It includes individual as well as collective traumata and refers to symptoms such as PTSD (Werner, 2020, p. 16). However, the origin of the term referred exclusively to a physical wound on the body. This idea of trauma being a shock has influenced its notion since at least the 17th century (Werner, 2020, p. 27).

Trauma is narrowly linked to memory. In the context of trauma art, Jill Bennett distinguishes 'common memory' and 'sense memory' (Bennett, 2005). In "common memory", experiences are processed through cognitive schemes and can be transformed into representation. The understanding that experiences can be represented at all has influenced trauma literature. Primarily informed by psychoanalysis, post-Holocaust theory and postmodernism, the traditional canon in trauma literature "defines trauma as unrepresentable and restricts its symbolization to an aesthetic of absence" (Werner, 2020, p. 11). According to Jill Bennett, the traumatic experience cannot be translated into a narrative, but it registers the physical imprint of the event. The art of sense memory enables a representational practice that generates sensations "so as to produce an encounter in the present" (Bennett, 2005, p. 28). Sense memory operates through the body to produce a kind of "seeing truth" and communicates a level of bodily affect (Bennett, 2005, p. 26). Bennett refers to a conception of art, not as aiming to reproduce the world (the Renaissance conception of art as representation), but as registering and producing affect, not as opposed to or distinct from thought, but as a means by which embodied understanding is produced (Bennett, 2005, p. 36). Art then

> . . . does not represent what has already occurred, but generates a set of aesthetic possibilities, which may in turn inform political thinking in regard to particular circumstances. If art can in some way evoke the pure event as a virtuality, the test is whether the virtual event is then amenable to different actualities.
>
> *(Bennett, 2012, p. 51)*

Sense memory aims to constitute a language of a subjective process to complement history and to work in a dialectical relationship with common memory. Anna-Lena Werner (2020), in her publication on how contemporary aesthetics challenge trauma as the unrepresentable, seeks

> . . . to legitimize artistic research and aesthetic practices as critical voices of a current public debate on trauma, as well as a tool of productivity for the active engagement in current conflicts and humanitarian and socio-political crises.
>
> *(Werner, 2020, p. 12)*

In recent years, and with the progress of various technologies, bringing about a reconsideration of the mechanisms of representation, the relationship between the image and reality has changed. From an artistic point of view, the image is not a representation, and truth, if there is any, lies in its material configuration. The image, as Hito Steyerl (2010) points out, "is a fragment of the real world. It is a thing just like any other – a thing like you and me." To participate in an image, then,

> . . . would mean participating in the material of the image as well as in the desires and forces it accumulates. How about acknowledging that this image is not some ideological misconception, but a thing simultaneously couched in affect and availability, a fetish made of crystals and electricity, animated by our wishes and fears – a perfect embodiment of its own conditions of existence? As such, the image is . . . without expression.

I am following the path of such understanding of the condition of the image, memory and traumatic events in the wider sense of the personal as well as the ecological and socio-political traumas that surround us. The traumas of circulating viruses, extreme drought and severe conflicts have become part of our daily lives. We have embodied them.

The four artistic positions explore memory and trauma in this wider sense. These are the Belgian artist Berlinde De Bruyckere, the American artist Matthew Barney, the Lithuanian artist Eglė Budvytytė and the Ukrainian artist and co-founder of FEMEN, Oksana Shachko. The different kinds of memories range from the cellular memory of the microbes in and around us to biographical and culturally embedded memories. Myth and religion play a significant role, whether explicit or implicit, embodied in the artists and their work. Trauma is never far away though. It is presented as an eco-political rather than a subjective phenomenon. In accordance with the central role that memory plays in the development of the body of work of each of the artists, it is significant that all of them can be linked to childhood memories with their special qualities. Children seem to show stronger memories for aspects that adults find rather unremarkable, such as, in my case, the flickering blue-green curtain that hung over the bed of the two-and-a-half-year-old. Such autobiographical memory can be understood less as semantic memory – or common memory, as Jill Bennett would say – but rather as a subtype of episodic memory (Nelson, 1993), referring to a complex process "which enables the retrieval of richly detailed evocative memories" (Irish & Piguet, 2013). They may translate into statements and manifests of artists later that can be seen as part of the artistic research (Varto, 2018). So, I will primarily let the artists speak. Their statements will be linked to concepts from scientific or literary fields and understood as analogies. According to the methodology of artistic (auto)ethnography, these fields build the contexts of the artistic awareness and the developing artworks.

Embalming affect: Berlinde De Bruyckere

Over several decades, Berlinde De Bruyckere has been working with casts of bodies, trees or horses, which she covers with fur or wax. The bodies are distorted in a way so that the horse's eyes are sewn up or human limbs are reconnected differently. They seem to be like hybrids of Greek torsos, barely living things that seek to escape their skin.

It is often mentioned that Berlinde De Bruyckere's father was a butcher which has influenced her work. But the artist sees it differently and more on the side of the working process:

> [My father. . .] was cutting dead animals into pieces to sell it, for people to eat. I do something very different. I take a dead body from the slaughterhouse . . . and bring it into my workshop, then I do all the modelling on the actual figure. It is as if I give the body a new life, so they can exist again because they have become a sculpture. I began asking myself what the most important thing was that I took from growing up surrounded by the dead animals and huge carcasses that I saw as a child. I think it is it that I am not afraid of dead bodies. I am used to seeing them . . . It was part of my childhood.
>
> *(De Bruyckere in Burley, 2012)*

Man of Sorrows

In 2006 Berlinde De Bruyckere exhibited *Man of Sorrows I and II*[1] at Kunsthalle Düsseldorf. It was the first time that she combined human and animal parts. Arms and stomachs are cast from horse limbs, whereas legs and feet come from a human model (Söntgen, 2006, p. 28). Once she had the moulds, Berlinde De Bruckere started adding layers of coloured wax to the mould. Finally, she joined the different parts of the body together to form the two sculptures. They are twisted around six-metre-high iron columns from an old, dilapidated railway station. It is no coincidence that the twisting of the bodies evokes the image of Christ at the whipping post. Growing up in Catholic surroundings in Ghent, some of the first pictures Berlinde De Bruyckere saw as a child were reproductions of paintings by Lucas Cranach the Elder. The artist feels an affinity with Cranach

> . . . because of the way he distorts the body. . . When I look at his paintings, I experience their physicality as the medium to express the thoughts and

> concerns of those figures: their fears, their passions, their doubts. . . It is all to do with man's mental state, which is evoked by the visible body.
>
> *(De Bruyckere in Theys, 2013)*

According to Jill Bennett's understanding of the togetherness of sense memory and common memory, religious images were not simply the 'Bible of the unlettered'. They conveyed the essence of Christ's sacrifice, the meaning of suffering, by promoting an empathetic imitation of Christ (Bennett, 2005). The operative element in the religious image is not the narrative framework but the affective detail – the wound (Schmid, 2015).

Phantom Limb Pain

Together with *Man of Sorrows*, Berlinde De Bruyckere showed a horse placed in a steel structure. The posture had been done with the help of special equipment that was installed for her in the Morphology Department of the Veterinary Faculty of Ghent University. The lifting apparatus helps to bring the animal's body into the correct position. Then silicon moulds are made. These moulds are cast in plaster and form the model for the work made from epoxy. The new formation of the body is made during this process (Söntgen, 2006, p. 15). Finally, the horse's body is covered with a new hide to make it whole again.

The togetherness of human and animal bodies in the exhibition links human and animal suffering. The conveyance of suffering through imagery and sculpture is possible as they have the capacity to address the spectator's own bodily memory, "to *touch* the viewer who *feels* rather than simply sees the event" (Bennett, 2005, p. 36).

The pain that might be evoked in the viewer by the horse's missing limbs can be linked to Phantom Limb Pain, the perception of pain in body regions that no longer exist. After extremity amputation, patients have often been reported to have painful sensations in missing limbs. Since the first record of Phantom Limb Pain (PLP) about a hundred years ago, thorough research has been conducted to figure out the pathophysiology of this phenomenon (Yixuan, 2020, p. 343). One possible attribution to PLP aetiology is the proprioceptive memory theory. According to this view, proprioceptive memory stands for the internal awareness and memory of limbs and their positions. Such a three-dimensional scheme is relatively independent and will not be affected by visual confirmation of an absent limb (Yixuan, 2020, p. 344). It is assumed the brain mechanisms that pertain to memory do not change.

> Because memories remain intact, proprioception occurs as it did prior to amputation. The realisation that a limb is missing arises through the visual

> system, but not the proprioception system. The rest of the body continues to work as it always has; nerves that are associated with the missing limb are still active.
>
> *(Weeks et al., 2010, p. 280)*

"The past is never dead. It's not even past", William Faulkner famously wrote.

Cats

"Cripplewood is not dead wood," John M. Coetzee wrote in the book accompanying Berlinde De Bruyckere's installation *Cripplewood-Kreupelhout* at the Venice Biennial in 2013 (Coetzee in Hirsch, 2013). After Berlinde De Bruyckere received the official news that she had been selected to represent Belgium she had, as is the tradition, to choose a curator to assist her during the artistic working process. Berlinde De Bruyckere preferred a different approach. She wrote to Coetzee:

> The last few months I buried myself in your work, and I draw so much of it . . . That is why I would like to ask you to be my curator. Not to . . . help make any decisions, but as a source of inspiration.
>
> *(De Bruyckere et al., 2013, p. 29)*

John answered:

> You suggest that . . . my role should be to provide new textual material for a joint publication. I attach a story that has not yet appeared in print . . . See what you think of it. I don't know what else I can suggest.
>
> *(Coetzee in De Bruyckere et al., 2013, p. 30)*

The story J.M. Coetzee sent was *The Old Woman and the Cats*. In the story, a son visits his mother who lives in the Spanish countryside feeding a dozen or more half feral cats. The cats, being everywhere in and around the house, function as a metaphor for letting things happen and by just letting things happen enabling them to live a life. The son asks his mother why she does not get the cats neutered so that the process of endless replication comes to an end. The mother replies:

> At the borders of being . . . there are all these small souls, cat souls, mouse souls, . . . souls of unborn children, crowded together, pleading to be let in, pleading to be incarnated. And I want to let them in, all of them, even if it is only for a day or two, even if it is only so that they can have a quick look at this beautiful world of ours. Because who am I to deny them their chance of incarnation?
>
> *(Coetzee in De Bruyckere et al., 2013, p. 23)*

Incarnated trees

Incarnation does not stop with humans and animals. In the last few decades, a lot of research has been done on the intelligence of plants. It is said that plants also have a drive to exist, "which is why they engage in complex, increasingly explored strategies of interaction with their environment and other species" (Frankfurter Kunstverein, 2021). They live in symbiosis, and I wish humankind was more aware that we all do. In the exhibition 'The Intelligence of Plants' at Frankfurter Kunstverein in 2021, Berlinde De Bruyckere exhibited two large oaks, *Embalmed Twins I and II*.[2] The artist tells how they came into being during a walk in a forest after Hurricane Cyrill in 2016:

> On a certain moment . . . I passed by two trees and they were down, . . . and what I saw was that one was still living and the other was already dead. So for me it was a very strange feeling looking to this choreography . . . And then I saw the bodies more than the trees. And that was a very important change in my mind to see them as bodies and not as trees anymore.
>
> *(De Bruyckere, 2022)*

Redoubt: Matthew Barney

Trees play a significant role in Matthew Barney's project *Redoubt*[3], developed from 2016 on. *Redoubt* includes a two-hour film that traces the story of a wolf hunt in Idaho's Sawtooth Mountain range, intertwining the theme of the hunt with those of mythology and artistic creation. The film is accompanied by five monumental sculptures, about fifty engravings and electroplated copper plates. The exhibition was first displayed at Yale University Art Gallery in 2019. *Redoubt* is, in a nutshell, the transformation of a mythological narrative into artistically embodied history.

Burning trees

For the catalogue, which is part of the project, Matthew Barney chose an article from 1899, *The Relation of Forests and Forest Fires* by Gifford Pinchot (Pinchot, 1899/2019). When Pinchot wrote his article the study of fires as modifiers of the composition of the forest was in its earliest stages (Pinchot, 1899/2019, p. 39). For Pinchot, there is no question that fires cause great damage, but the focus of his article is the regulative action of fire on the forest. Perhaps the most remarkable of the regulative effects of forest fires relates to the kinds of trees of which it is composed and the proportion of each. This effect depends on the qualities of resistance which trees possess. These qualities are of two chief kinds: one, adapted to secure the safety of the individual tree, the other to assure the continuance of the species, with little regard for the single tree.

An example of the first kind is the western larch, whose enormously thick bark is almost fireproof. In young trees, the bark is often as thick as the wood and individuals may reach an age of three or four thousand years (Pinchot, 1899/2019, p. 43). The second method of protection against fire is used by thin-barked trees like the lodgepole pine. This results from the hoarding of the ripe seeds in the cones for several years. Fire kills the standing tree and leaves it to be blown down years after when decay will have weakened the roots. In the meantime, the hoarded winged seeds are set free by the opening of the cones, are then distributed and germinate.

Matthew Barney spent a lot of time in forest fire areas in Idaho and

> . . . started seeing these trees and the different character, from tree to tree. Some of that plays out in the film, but it was starting to play out in my head – in the sculptures that could come out of that.
>
> *(Barney, 2021)*

The artistic process led to the incarnation of fire. Barney extracted some of the trees from those burn regions, brought them to his workshop, and with the help of a computer-driven mill made a mould out of them. Hot liquid metal was poured inside the tree. Barney combined different metals in order to marbleise them. In the piece "Elk Creek Burn", made from a lodgepole pine, we see at the end, where the metal exits the tree, a kind of fins, which:

> . . . are something like the positive of what you would see in a burned tree, which would be the negative cracks. I think it was an attempt to try to capture some of the energy of these burned trees and the sort of trauma that they've been exposed to.
>
> *(Barney, 2021)*

The transformative quality of fire functions both as a metaphor and as a means of artistic experimentation. It was this level of experimentation that Barney wanted to carry through the whole body of work. According to Jill Bennett, such experimental artistic language finds expression in that which is beyond representation (Bennett, 2005, p. 15).

Diana and the wolves in Idaho

That also counts for the film *Redoubt*, where Barney experimented with movements in order to develop an embodied instead of a spoken language. The plot is loosely attached to the ancient myth of Diana – a virgin goddess and patroness of the hunter and the moon – and Actaeon, a young hunter. The narrative is transposed to the remote wilderness of Idaho's Sawtooth Mountains. Diana is played by a professional sharpshooter and Barney himself acts as Actaeon – not as a hunter of animals but as an engraver of perceptions.

The myth of Diana and Actaeon stems from Ovid's *Metamorphoses*. The tale recounts the fate of a young hunter and his encounter with Diana. The latter is nude and enjoying a bath in a spring with help from her escort of nymphs when the mortal man unwittingly appears. The nymphs scream in surprise and attempt to cover Diana, who, embarrassed, splashes water upon Actaeon. He is transformed into a deer, robbed of his ability to speak, and flees in fear.

The nymphs in *Redoubt* are dancers and no one talks. During the production, Barney looked at a lot of historical paintings of Diana and the dead animals next to her and linked these aesthetic experiences to certain aspects of wildlife management and land management in the area. It seemed to him "like the choices that were made a long time ago that we sort of carry forward" (Barney, 2019b). To Barney, the character of Diana felt important in view of transposing the ancient myth into the 1980s when he was growing up in Central Idaho. At that time wolves had been a significant topic because the state of Idaho had decided to reintroduce them into the mountains. The debate in the following years was quite controversial and illuminated the political divide of society. What kept Barney's imagination was:

> . . . just how the argument around the reintroduction of the wolf itself had a kind of mythological scale to it, that it wasn't really about the issues that people were talking about, it was bigger than that and so I kept coming back to it.
>
> *(Barney, 2019b)*

The artist wanted to deal with the political situation with the wolves without making a political work. He wanted to approach the subject aesthetically, and this is what *Redoubt* is all about.

Alchemy

Matthew Barney dealt with the engravings he made during the filming process in a similar way to the artistic experimentation with trees and movements. The copper plates were covered with asphalt so that the needle would break that surface. The plates were dropped into a bath of sulfuric acid. Copper, Barney explains, is in suspension in that bath and through an electrochemical reaction the copper is:

> . . . attracted to an opposite pole of electricity that's connected to the plate. It gravitates toward that engraved line and it builds up and becomes a positive where there was a negative and it keeps growing.
>
> *(Barney, 2019b)*

Barney considers this material transformation an integral part of the story (Barney, 2021). One might say that this is the alchemist aspect in his work. It is illuminated in a scene near the beginning of the film when Barney and the Electroplater dig up a copper plate from the soil outside of the caravan where the electroplating process takes place. In one of the last scenes of the movie, wolves enter the caravan, tear bed sheets apart, drink the sulfuric acid bath and bring the artistic results back to nature where they came from.

Singing soil: Eglė Budvytytė

The costumes that the Lithuanian artist Eglė Budvytytė used in her 2020 film, *Songs from the Compost: Mutating Bodies, Imploding Stars*,[4] literally came from soil. They were made by the artist's collaborators Marija Olšauskaitė and Julija Steponaitytė through composting the fabrics. The clothes have been dug into the soil where they rotted and were partly eaten by microorganisms and bacteria. So the costumes act as metaphors for beyond human embodiment. They reverberate the central ideas of the film: that of dying and decay. The film was created from songs, written and performed by Eglė Budvytytė. They are, as she writes in her artist book, "love letters" to the novelist Octavia E. Butler and to the biologist Lynn Margulis (Budvytytė, 2020). The lyrics in the song *Bacteria and Time* draw from ideas of the latter, addressing the role of bacteria in making life possible and the collaboration between the one-cell organisms:

> how about
> decay, rotting, decomposing
> as technologies for non-linear time
> . . .
> bacteria
> will take care of you
> . . .
> she'll fuck your past
> she'll set you loose
> she'll digest you.
>
> *(Budvytytė, 2020)*

Bacteria and time

"Look into my shapeless eyes," bacteria sings in her song. To read Margulis is:

> . . . to become acquainted with different bacteria merging together . . . . Reading [her] is like re-writing the inherited visions of gender, time, humanness, individuality and opening up to other ways of sensing and seeing things.
>
> *(Budvytytė, 2020)*

About two decades ago, Lynn Margulis addressed symbiosis as the crucial momentum of evolution. The very cells we are made of started as symbiotic unions of different kinds of bacteria. That we see microbes and bacteria as enemy agents stems, in the eyes of Margulis, from taxonomy, from naming the living (Margulis, 1998, p. 70). She sees language and fixed categorisations as misconceptions that lead to the assumption that all bacteria should be eradicated. Margulis tries to replace this, "oversimplified cultural nonsense with concepts . . . closer to . . . scientific descriptions" (Margulis, 1998, p. 71).

Margulis' concept was not recognised in her time. It very much clashed with the classical biological view of life and the individual. In the early modern period the appearance of the independent citizen, "mirroring the notion of the autonomous individual agent framed a biology that was organised around the study of particulate, interacting, living entities" (Gilbert, 2012, p. 326). In the Darwinian view of life, individuals are identifiable units in competition with one another. Cells were understood as agents, constructing autonomous organisms. This view became a frame for the formulation of social normativity, and

> . . . leads either to misinterpreting or simply missing a large amount of biological diversity. Nature is then used as a comparison to human sociality and sexuality, and, consequently, non-normative practices, identities, and communities lose out – reframed as necessarily unnatural.
>
> *(Griffiths, 2015, p. 42)*

With Margulis' concept, the classical view on individuals was challenged and symbiosis became a core principle of contemporary biology. It started to replace an essentialist conception of individuality. Her "findings lead us into directions that transcend the self/nonself, subject/object dichotomies that have characterized Western thought" (Gilbert *et al.*, 2012, p. 326).

The first cells in our lineage were self-maintaining systems. Surprisingly, they very much resemble us: "The insides of our bodies today are chemically more akin to the external environment of the early Earth . . . than they are like our present . . . world" (Margulis, 1998, p. 108). Our symbiogenetic composite core is far older than the recent innovation we call the individual human (Margulis, 1998, p. 124). Life is cyclical insofar as a memory-storing system. It is, as Margulis puts it, a series of selves, whether organisms or cells. These need energy to continue to exist, and they do so in an unseverable connection to past life. "Life has been, since inception and with no discontinuity, chemically connected to its past" (Margulis, 1998, p. 101). The past is never dead.

Proprioception

Eglė Budvytytė sees *Songs from the Compost* as a performance of "how things seamlessly are dying and growing at the same time" (Budvytytė, 2021, 05:37).

This is mirrored by the body weight and the surrendering of the bodies to each other and the forest floor. The choreography is based on proprioception. It echoes the idea of beyond the human embodiment in the way the bodies engage with the landscape in a more horizontal than vertical way (Budvytytė, 2021, 04:40). Proprioception is probably as old as life itself. The Earth has, according to Lynn Margulis, "enjoyed a proprioceptive system for millennia, since long before humans evolved. Small mammals communicate the coming earthquake . . . Trees release . . . substances that warn their neighbours that gypsy moth larvae are attacking their leaves" (Margulis, 1998, 141f). Even viruses communicate on a chemical level. It was only in 2017 that a team of microbiologists from Weizmann Institute of Science in Israel found that some bacteriophages – viruses that infect bacteria – communicate via the encoding of peptides to decide if they go on killing their hosts or to let them stay alive. Apparently, the bacteriophages thus use a feedback mechanism to regulate the number of bacterial hosts to ensure optimum availability for newly formed viruses (Erez *et al.*, 2017).

The forest

Eglė Budvytytė employs movements and songs to address the relationship between bodies and their environment, and the permeable boundaries between the human and non-human. The film was shot in the forests and sand dunes of the Curonian Spit, in an environment where the lichen, a symbiotic composite organism formed by algae and fungi, is present everywhere. In the lichen, the green algae themselves photosynthesise through their chloroplasts, which are ancestral symbiotic cyanobacteria. This is symbiosis within symbioses, symbionts all the way down (Griffiths, 2015, p. 39). All individuals are chimeric. Thinking with lichens then can "offer a queer way out of heteronormative narratives of human and non-human sexuality and sociality by decentering heterosexual biological reproduction as the *only* way that life (re) produces" (Griffiths, 2015, p. 39).

The film premiered in the exhibition *The Spectral Forest* at Nida Art Colony; that is in the context of the histories of deforestation and afforestation on the Curonian Spit. For the Curonians, a tribe inhabiting the shores of the Baltic Sea until the sixteenth century, and after whom the spit was named, sacred groves were closely associated with the cult of the dead. In the 1970s, folk traditions were mobilised against Soviet industrial, secular modernity which dismissed most spiritual culture as regressive (Ištok, 2021).

The exhibition took place within the context of the European Cooperation Project 4Cs: From Conflict to Conviviality through Creativity and Culture. So, connectivity is a crucial moment. On the Curonian Spit, connectivity takes many shapes. One could think of the root systems of the forest linked by fungi, their mycelia acting as a kind of underground internet (Ištok, 2021). This points to

Donna Haraway's (2008) hypotheses that the biological and the social are always interconnected, challenging the bridge between what counts as nature and what counts as culture. So, the view of the individual as a symbiont that cannot be seen separate from everything else has consequences for the view on sociality and bio-politics.

Gaia

We all are embedded in the larger context of the Earth as a network of ecosystems (Margulis, 1998, p. 133). Around 1996 the question arose as to whether all life on the planet constituted a superorganism and if life was one single self-regulating entity called Gaia. The author of the Gaia hypothesis was James Lovelock. The term was suggested to Lovelock by the novelist William Golding. Lovelock asked his then neighbour whether he could replace the phrase "a cybernetic system with homeostatic tendencies as detected by chemical anomalies in the Earth's atmosphere" with a "good four-letter word", as he said. Golding suggested Gaia, the ancient Greek word for "Mother Earth" (Margulis, 1998, p. 147f). Gaia was meant as a "name for an Earthwide phenomenon: the regulation of temperature . . . and gas composition" (Margulis, 1998, p. 150). But soon "religiously inclined people, attracted to the idea of a native goddess with power . . . giving Gaia a distinctly non-scientific connotation" (Margulis, 1998, p. 148). Lynn Margulis regrets this personification. Gaia is not an organism but the regulated surface of the planet incessantly creating new environments and organisms.

Ikonoclasts: Oksana Shachko

The disappointment of a non-existing god in a brutal political environment was the origin of Oksana Shachko's interest in activist politics. She was born in 1987 in Ukraine in the city of Khmelnitsky. In the same year, the first unit of the Khmelnitsky Power Plant became operational. Oksana Shachko's family was very religious, so a certain social tension accompanied her from the very beginning, as she explains in an interview in 2017 (Leturcq & Shachko, 2017). When she was eight years old, Oksana Shachko's parents sent her to an iconography school. She learnt all the antique techniques of traditional icon painting – working with wood, gold and different metals. But Oksana Shachko learnt not only about the techniques but also about how icons are codified – the symbols that need to be copied in a careful and accurate way. To live in the world of icons had a huge influence on the child:

> I was deeply inside the religious world and very concentrated on my craft. . . . At ten years old I had already started painting in churches and exhibiting

> my art. I was deeply inside all these institutional bodies, and because of it, I started believing in God . . . When I was twelve years old I decided to go live in the church, to paint icons and spend my life praying. I wanted to stop living a normal life and become a monk.
>
> *(Leturcq & Shachko, 2017)*

She was about to marry Jesus, and it came to her as a big surprise that her parents saw this as a tragedy. She did not want to overwhelm them with stress and decided to stay. But from then on Oksana Shachko started to think about the meaning of believing: "I continued painting icons but started engaging in more conversations with the people surrounding me. I wanted to know why they came and prayed in front of these icons" (Leturcq & Shachko, 2017).

At the age of 14, Oksana Shachko found a group of young people who organised philosophical clubs. They were very critical of religion. She discussed religion with them and wanted to prove it to them. In vain. After a few years, she became

> . . . a total atheist. Finally, I understood there was no place for God in life. . . . I understood that religion is just a fucking business and a tool to manipulate society. That made me very angry and I stopped painting the icons.
>
> *(Leturcq & Shachko, 2017)*

FEMEN, a radical feminist group, was created and Oksana Shacho started to use performance as a way to fight. After emigrating to Paris and leaving FEMEN in 2014, she started painting icons again and called them *Iconoclasts*. With the icons, she continued FEMEN's fights against "the sex industry . . . against dictatorships and all the religions" (Leturcq & Shachsko, 2017) just in another medium. Her first solo exhibition in 2016 took place at the Galerie Mansart in Paris.[5]

In the paintings the manufacturing protocol is perfectly respected: preparing the wooden panels, painting with tempera, laying gold leaves and respecting the historical choreography of the icons. But Virgo lactans, the traditional motif of the nursing Mary, now wears a burka. The archangel Michael, Horseman of the Apocalypse, becomes a woman rider. She used one of the most famous icons, Andreï Roublev's Holy Trinity, several times as a blueprint for her fight. What was understood as the embodiment of spiritual unity, peace, harmony, mutual love and humility in Roublev's time, is transformed into three angels smoking and drinking, wearing masks and wearing niqabs. The furniture is drawn in reverse, respectively multiple perspectives and thus addressed to a pre- or post-human subject. The viewer can easily imagine that the angels rise and leave nothing but a golden space and the structure of empty chairs. Empty chairs, this is what is left. The icons and part of their coming into being through the painting process can still be seen on the artist's Instagram page which remains active after her death in July 2018.

Remembering the body

"I want to know how we represent with the body in movement," said choreographer William Forsythe (Forsythe after Brandtstetter *et al.*, 2000, p. 16). This question is inseparably connected with body memory and with remembering the body, understood as reaching further than our mere skin.

In the cultural and religious tradition of Christian art, the spiritual takes the place of the corporeal. This is the tradition in which Oksana Shachko made an icon out of herself.

> We used art to talk about bigger problems. As an iconographer . . . I wanted to make iconic images of our movement. After two years of figuring it out, I think I managed to create this image: the girl with a flower crown in her hair, the strong positions with the fist up and straight legs, the slogans on the body and the angry face. It's a lot of work to put all those details together.
>
> *(Shachko in Leturcq, 2017)*

The Christian tradition, and the fact that she grew up in a post-Soviet city, led Oksana Shachko to embody icons and to represent her political engagement through the means of a spiritual medium, which is what the icon in Christianity is.

Body and motion memory is what interests Eglė Budvytytė in her work. In her songs about bacteria and human animals she looks at rhythm and the hypnotic effect that it could cause (Budvytytė, 2021, 08:39).

> I've been interested in trauma for a while, and the visceral effect of voice onto the nervous system of the receiver. When I sing or when I record, I try to have that in the back of my brain, how these sounds will be massaging the nervous system of the receiver.
>
> *(Budvytytė, 2021, 07:52)*

This points out to dis-membering and re-membering – a concept that Gabriele Brandstetter used for describing the decomposition and reconstruction of bodies in choreography as well as in myth and culture (Brandstetter *et al.*, 2000, p. 18f). Dis-membering in myth and religion includes violence, destruction, pain and loss.

The double nature of memory as disintegration and reconstruction is mirrored in Matthew Barney's film *Redoubt*. The myth of Diana was a key for him to be able to maintain some kind of balance for himself (Barney, 2019b). On a shelf we see books about mythology, wolves, the universe and Bonnie Bainbridge Cohen's approach to embodiment and movement analysis. The hints to his research are paralleled with the artistic development of the first sculpture that Barney made entirely of wood, using the trunk of a tree felled in Idaho.

Barney combines traditional carving with digital editing techniques. "The trauma of the burnt forest is evident in the scarred surface of the tree, where carved-out wounds . . . evoke associations with medieval religious wooden sculptures" (Hetzler, 2021).

The way Berlinde De Bruyckere wants to frame her work is that there is always a certain duality between pain and healing (De Bruyckere, 2015). For Coetzee's story *The Old Woman and the Cats* fits so perfectly. The woman not only feeds cats in her house in order to help all the unborn souls to come in but also gives room for a mentally disabled man whom she saves from being committed to an asylum. Berlinde De Bruyckere's embalmed trees can be seen as reminiscent of the concept of the body in ancient Egypt, where memory is transformed through embalming rituals. It is not the living body that is the focus of attention, but rather the body that is produced after death. "Cripplewood is alive," Coetzee wrote (Coetzee after Hirsch, 2013).

Trauma and the queer nature of lichen

If trauma enters the representational arena as an expression of personal experience, it is always vulnerable to appropriation, reduction and mimicry. The art of trauma must be something other than the deposit of primary experiences that remain unshareable, even if communicated (Bennett, 2005, p. 6). The experiences art offers do not invite us to extrapolate a persona from them. "The affective responses engendered by artworks are not born of emotional identification or sympathy; rather they emerge from a direct engagement with sensation as it is registered in the work" (Bennett, 2005, p. 7).

Art in arts therapies is not a vehicle for interpersonal transmission of experience but rather embodies the ability to transform our perception. It is, as John Dewey put it, the moral function of art "to remove prejudice, to do away with the scales that keep the eye from seeing, tear away the veils due to wont and custom, perfect the power to perceive" (Dewey, 1934/1980, p. 325). A synopsis of artistic practice and arts-therapeutic practice becomes apparent when we realise that arts therapists always act in the different roles of artist, therapist and often researcher. The subject-based generation of knowledge that the professional artistic practice offers is relevant to arts therapists, understood as reflective practitioners, with regard to the further development of artistic-therapeutic interventions.

Art may open us up to phenomena like the symbiotic nature of lichen. The concept of symbiosis can be relevant for arts therapies (education) as it – in accordance with the biopsychosocial model – challenges health practices and other regulatory mechanisms. If we view all bodies as multispecies assemblages rather than as either clean, healthy and pure or infected, unhealthy and impure, this view "could thus have consequences for how infected bodies are conceived of, and therefore treated and cared for" (Griffiths, 2015, p. 38). If bodies are recognised as always already inhabited by countless bacteria and viruses, then this could potentially alleviate the social stigma that accompanies certain illnesses and conditions.

> If heteronormativity . . . no longer define[s] the frame through which nature is viewed, then this will have an effect on the definition of some social and cultural practices as 'natural'. This is important politically, as normativity masquerading as nature necessarily supports the conservative status quo and is hostile to non-normativity. Queer theory for lichens suggests that we have never been individuals, and that attention to this can have positive biomedical consequences.
>
> *(Griffiths, 2015, p. 44)*

The queer nature of lichen and its inextricable link to the past can influence the politics of arts therapies and the way memory as a beyond- human phenomenon is dealt with. The image is a thing like you and me.

Notes

1 For images see: https://www.hauserwirth.com/hauser-wirth-exhibitions/2901-berlinde-bruyckere-schmerzensmann/ (accessed 17 September 2023).
2 For images see: https://www.fkv.de/berlinde-de-bruyckere/ (accessed 17 September 2023).
3 For images and trailer see: https://grasshopperfilm.com/film/redoubt/ and https://artgallery.yale.edu/exhibitions/exhibition/matthew-barney-redoubt (accessed 17 September 2023).
4 For images see: https://www.eglebudvytyte.lt/songs-from-the-compost-mutating-bodies-imploding-stars/ (accessed 17 September 2023).
5 For images see: https://www.galerie-mansart.fr/expos/iconoclaste-oksana-schachko and https://www.instagram.com/oksanashachko/?hl=de (accessed 17 September 2023).

References

Barney, M., Franks, P., Hodermarsky, E. and Wiles, S. (2019). *Matthew Barney: Redoubt*. New Haven: Yale University Art Gallery.

Barney, M. (2019a). ActionMedia TALK Matthew Barney: Redoubt/UCCA. [Video]. *YouTube*. Available at: https://www.youtube.com/watch?v=Ff8BI5ijLt8&t=146s (accessed 23 August 2022).

Barney, M. (2019b). FF Presents: REDOUBT – Matthew Barney, 30 October 2019. [Video] *YouTube*. Available at: https://www.youtube.com/watch?v=lP2YuzsIBoo&t=301s (accessed 23 August 2022).

Barney, M. (2021). Matthew Barney on his Redoubt exhibition at Hayward Gallery, June 2021. [Video] *YouTube*. Available at: https://www.youtube.com/watch?v=Ad7QvjPlYCM (accessed 23 August 2022).

Bennett, J. (2005). *Empathic Vision. Affect, Trauma, and Contemporary Art*. Stanford: Stanford University Press.

Bennett, J. (2012). *Practical Aesthetics. Events, Affects and Art after 9/11*. London and New York: I.B. Tauris.

Brandstetter, G. (2000). Choreography As a Cenotaph: The Memory of Movement. In *ReMembering the Body*. Körper-Bilder in Bewegung, (eds). v. Gabriele Brandstetter and Hortensia Völckers, mit Stress, einem Bildessay von Bruce Mau mit Texten von André Lepecki. Ostfildern-Ruit: Hatje Cantz.
Budvytytė, E. with Marija Olšauskaitė and Julija Steponaitytė, Songs from the Compost: Mutating Bodies, Imploding Stars, 2020. HD video, 29 min. Commissioned for The Spectral Forest, NAC of Vilnius Academy of Arts within the framework of 4Cs and 2nd Riga International Biennial of Contemporary Art, RIBOCA2. Photo by Ansis Starks.
Budvytytė, E. (2020). *Songs from the Compost*. PDF artist book by Eglė Budvytytė. Vilnius: The Baltic Notebooks of Anthony Blunt.
Budvytytė, E. (2020a). Songs from the compost. Mutating bodies, exploding stars. Available at: https://www.eglebudvytyte.lt/songs-from-the-compost-mutating-bodies-imploding-stars/ (accessed 29 May 2023).
Budvytytė, E. (2021). Lithuanian Visual Artists: Eglė Budvytytė. 30.11.2021. Presentation in Lithuanian Culture Institute. [Video] *YouTube*. Available at: https://www.youtube.com/watch?v=tsL-u6CRWng&t=562s (accessed 28 August 2022).
Burley, I. (2012). Berlinde De Bruyckere: Three Sculptures. Interview with Berlinde De Bruyckere. In: *AnOther*, 4 December 2012. https://www.anothermag.com/art-photography/2376/berlinde-de-bruyckere-three-sculptures (accessed 19 August 2022)
De Bruyckere, B., Coetzee, J.M. and van Cauteren, P. (2013). *Cripplewood = Kreupelhout*. Brussels: Mercatorfonds.
De Bruyckere, B. (2015). The Embalmer, Kunsthaus Bregenz & Kunstraum Dornbirn. [Video] *YouTube*. Available at: https://www.youtube.com/watch?v=Wl0jR_vnLvU&list=PLusTeaHXQKaDhPwIwDOzhgNOrtWWn9hUv&index=62&t=45s (accessed 10 May 2023).
De Bruyckere, B. (2022). Die Intelligenz der Pflanzen. Frankfurter Kunstverein. [Video] *YouTube*. Available at: https://www.youtube.com/watch?v=K2marxih9Pg (accessed 30 August 2022).
Dewey, J. (1934/1980). *Art as Experience*. New York: Perigee Printing.
Erez, Z., Steinberger-Levy, I., Shamir, M. *et al.* (2017). Communication between viruses guides lysis–lysogeny decisions. *Nature* 541, 488–493. https://doi.org/10.1038/nature21049
Faulkner, W. (1951). *Requiem for a Nun*. New York: Penguin Random House.
Frankfurter Kunstverein. (2021). The Intelligence of Plants. Available at: https://www.fkv.de/ausstellung/die-intelligenz-der-pflanzen/ (accessed 30 August 2022).
Galerie Mansart. (2016). Iconoclaste. Oksana Schachko. 12 May–19 June 2016; Vernissage: 12 mai 2016 18:00–22:00. Commissariat: Azad Asifovich. Available at: https://www.galerie-mansart.fr/expos/iconoclaste-oksana-schachko (accessed 24 August 2022).
Galerie Max Hetzler (2021). *Matthew Barney: After Ruby Ridge*. Exhibition from 14 September–23 December 2021. Available at: https://www.maxhetzler.com/exhibitions/matthew-barney-2021/press-de/ (accessed 24 May 2023).
Gilbert, S.F., Sapp, J. and Tauber, A.I. (2012). A Symbiotic View of Life: We Have Never Been Individuals. *The Quarterly Review of Biology*, 87(4), December, 325–341. Available at: https://www.jstor.org/stable/10.1086/668166 (accessed 24 May 2023).
Griffiths, D. (2015). Queer Theory for Lichens. *UnderCurrents: Journal of Critical Environmental Studies*, 19, 36–45. https://doi.org/10.25071/2292-4736/40249 (accessed 24 May 2023).
Haraway, D.J. (2008). *When Species Meet*. Posthumanities 3. Minneapolis: University of Minnesota Press.
Hirsch, F. (2013). Correspondences: An Interview with Berlinde De Bruyckere. *Art News*, 2 July 2013. Available at: https://www.artnews.com/art-in-america/interviews/correspondences-an-interview-with-berlinde-de-bruyckere-56331/ (accessed 9 September 2022).

Irish, M. & Piguet, O. (2013). The Pivotal Role of Semantic Memory in Remembering the Past and Imagining the Future. *Frontiers in Behavioral Neuroscience*, 7. https://www.frontiersin.org/articles/10.3389/fnbeh.2013.00027 doi: 10.3389/fnbeh.2013.00027 (accessed 9 May 2023).

Ištok, R. (2021). Introduction to the Catalogue the Spectral Forest. In Rado Ištok (ed.), *The Spectral Forest*. Vilnius: Nida Art Colony of the Vilnius Academy of Arts.

Leturcq, A. & Shachko, O. (2017). A Meeting between Oksana Shachko and Armelle Leturcq. [Interview]. Available at: https://www.crash.fr/a-meeting-with-oksana-shachko/ (accessed 12 March 2022).

Liu, Y. (2020). The Pathophysiology of Phantom Limb Pain. In *Advances in Social Science, Education and Humanities Research*, Volume 496, Proceedings of the 2020 3rd International Conference on Humanities Education and Social Sciences (ICHESS 2020).

Mambrol, N. (2018). Trauma Studies. *Literary Theory and Criticism*. Available at: https://literariness.org/2018/12/19/trauma-studies/ (accessed 9 May 2023).

Margulis, L. (1998). *Symbiotic Planet: A New Look at Evolution*, 1st edn. Science masters. New York: Basic Books.

Nelson, K. (1993). The Psychological and Social Origins of Autobiographical Memory. *Psychological Science*, 4(1), 7–14.

Pinchot, G. (1899/2019). The Relation of Forests and forest Fires. In M. Barney, P. Franks, E. Hodermarsky and S. Wiles (2019), *Matthew Barney: Redoubt*. New Haven: Yale University Art Gallery.

Schmid, G. (2015). Die Architektur der Erinnerung. Künstlermythos und Vermittlungsstrategien in den autobiographischen Schriften von Louise Bourgeois. In B. Böckem, O. Peters and B. Schellewald (eds), *Die Biographie – Mode oder Universalie? Zu Geschichte und Konzept einer Gattung in der Kunstgeschichte*. Schriften zur modernen Kunsthistoriographie 7. Berlin: De Gruyter.

Shachko, O. oksanashachko. *Instagram*. Available at: https://www.instagram.com/oksanashachko/?hl=de (accessed 11 May 2023).

Söntgen, B. (2006). Hide and Hair. Berlinde De Bruyckere's Art of Envisioning. In Kunsthalle Düsseldorf (eds), *under cover – aus dem Verborgenen. Berlinde De Bruyckere Martin Honert*. Catalogue. Köln: Walter König.

Steyerl, H. (2010). A Thing Like You and Me. *eflux Journal*, 15(April 2010). Available at: https://www.e-flux.com/journal/15/61298/a-thing-like-you-and-me/

Theys, H. (2008). Berlinde De Bruyckere – 2008 – Over sokkels voor de nacht en over verzachtende omstandigheden. Available at: http://hanstheys.ensembles.org/ensembles/text-material?item=16561&locale=de&panel=113 (accessed 15 May 2023).

Theys, H. (2013). A conversation with Berlinde De Bruyckere. *Arte y Pensamiento Con temporáneo*, 24 November 2013. Available at: https://arteypensamientocontemporaneo.wordpress.com/2013/11/24/hans-theys-a-conversation-with-berlinde-de-bruyckere/ (accessed 20 August 2022).

Varto, J. (2018). *Artistic Research: What Is It? Who Does It? Why?* Aalto University Publication Series. Art + Design + Architecture 6/2018. Espoo: Aalto University, School of Arts, Design and Architecture, Department of Arts.

Weeks, S.R., Anderson-Barnes, V.C. and Tsao, J.W. (2010). Phantom Limb Pain: Theories and Therapies. In *The Neurologist*, 16(5), September. doi: 10.1097/NRL.0b013e3181edf128

Werner, A. (2020). *Let Them Haunt Us: How Contemporary Aesthetics Challenge Trauma as the Unrepresentable*. Bielefeld: transcript Verlag.

4

THE ARTIST AS AEDO

Memory, Absence and Materiality

Marián Cao

Abstract

Tzvetan Todorov (2000) distinguishes two types of memory, a literal and an exemplary one. As opposed to a way of interpreting the past as unique and unrepeatable – literal memory – Todorov proposes an exemplary memory, which recalls that past and turns it into a principle of action for the present. Memory, the present of the past, sets the debate on the future in tension. At the same time, trauma, as a memory where the past does not move forwards, remains stuck in a frozen time where forgiveness becomes impossible. This chapter aims to address how art, through its materiality and processes, activates exemplary memory, mobilises the void on the one hand, and matter, the material redoubt of the world, as a metaphor for transformation, on the other hand.

The artist then recovers the function of the Greek aedo. Aedos (from the Greek ἀοιδός, *aoidós*, singer) were, in Ancient Greece, artists who sang epics collected from the population and shaped into lyrics. These artists, whose process we present and analyse in this chapter, aedos of the memory of the vanquished, collect the strands of the memory of pain, recompose them, giving them materiality and exhibiting them so that they can be shared. They are thus necessary vehicles of social mourning.

I have chosen three artists: Gustavo Germano or showing absence; Art al Quadrat, or hair as a vestige of the body and stigma; Doris Salcedo, or steel as a symbol of transformation and water as (dis)appearance.

Through the absence of material transformation, the three artists bring together the action of the community, uniting the intimate and the common, facilitating

DOI: 10.4324/9781032663944-4

a social elaboration and grief, which, as a form of community art therapy, demands social recognition and contributes to the construction of an exemplary memory that affects the present.

Keywords: aedo, memory, forgiveness, mourning, art, art therapy

Abstract in Spanish

Tzvetan Todorov (2000) distingue dos tipos de memoria, una literal y otra ejemplar. Frente a una forma de interpretar el pasado como único e irrepetible – la memoria literal-, Todorov propone una memoria ejemplar, que recupera ese pasado y lo convierte en principio de acción para el presente. La memoria, presente del pasado, pone en tensión el debate sobre el futuro. A la vez, el trauma, como memoria donde el pasado no avanza, queda prendido en un tiempo congelado donde el perdón se hace imperdonable. Este capítulo pretende abordar cómo el arte, a través de su materialidad y sus procesos, activa la memoria ejemplar, moviliza el vacío, por un lado, y la materia, reducto de materialidad del mundo, como metáfora de transformación, por otro.

El artista recupera entonces la función del aedo griego. Los aedos (del griego ἀοιδός, aoidós, "cantor") eran, en la Antigua Grecia, artistas que cantaban epopeyas recogidas entre la población y plasmadas en letras. Estos artistas, cuyo proceso presentamos y analizamos en este capítulo, aedos de la memoria de los vencidos, recogen los hilos de la memoria del dolor, los recomponen, les dan materialidad y los exponen para que puedan ser compartidos. Son así vehículos necesarios del duelo social.

Hemos elegido a tres artistas: Gustavo Germano, o mostrar la ausencia; Art al Quadrat, o el cabello como vestigio del cuerpo y estigma; Doris Salcedo, o el acero como símbolo de transformación y el agua como desaparición.

A través de la ausencia o la transformación material, los tres artistas aglutinan la acción de la comunidad, uniendo lo íntimo y lo común, facilitando una elaboración social y un duelo que, como forma de arteterapia comunitaria, exige el reconocimiento social y contribuye a la construcción de una memoria ejemplar que incide en el presente.

The memory of matter

I was renovating the bathroom at my home. In just one day, a tiled, smooth and polished bathroom was turned into debris. How quick destruction operates. When Fernando, the architect, arrived, I went with him into what was now suddenly a small space of rubble. A space revealing walls where you could guess the history of a 19th-century house through the materials that emerged: handmade brick, cracked wood, crumbling cement, ropes that seemed to be damp, emerging from somewhere dark, ready to vanish when you touched them. I commented to Fernando, looking around, "It gives the impression that it's all a lie". He looked at me with astonishment and curiosity, "What's a lie?" And I told him, as we both inhaled the tiny particles of dust that entered our noses and pores, amidst the fragments that we were discovering before our eyes like strata of a freshly cut mountain, that the reality we were used to, of smooth, homogeneous, closed and clean porcelain, concealed all this: disused materials, some of them degraded, a strange amalgam of tones, smells, textures and diverse origins that enveloped us. And that, in everyday life, there was a lie that concealed all this. He looked at my arm and said to me, "Since when is skin a lie?" And I looked at my arm in turn and the two of us began to talk about organs, blood and viscera. As much a lie or as true as the skin that covers us.

The last and the current century have brought a paradigm shift in our relationship with the world. Vision has replaced all other senses. We have subordinated hearing, which we used to listen to our own words as we read aloud and that now we silence – as Irene Vallejo (2021) well recounts in *El infinito en un junco* – and we have ceased to be attentive to the signs of nature and the murmur of the seasons. The Covid-19 pandemic has made us frightened of touch and contact, the support of the first relationship with our maternal and paternal referent, the place of caress or pain, that body that "keeps count" as Bessel Van der Kolk (2015) points out, that preserves the imprint of the relationship with others, and awakens the capacity to feel, by touching, the roughness, the humidity, the softness, the warmth, the cold or the wrinkle. Smell, that necessary and forgotten sense that has the capacity to inform us, to move us and transform us, has been invaded, if not replaced by the gaze, the image and its perception. All computer gadgets focus on the flat vision of our knowledge of the world. We have forgotten how all the other senses – smell, taste, the sensation of dampness, spatiality, the touch of objects – informed us about the world. We even reduce ourselves to the flatscreen image of the mobile phone to know who we are. The written word, looked at on paper and read in solitude, is no longer the voice pronounced in the community. Situational thinking has been replaced by abstract thinking, in the words of Walter Ong (1982), and whispered words by a signifying concept that encloses content without matter.

Juhani Pallasmaa (2021) in his excellent work *The Eyes of the Skin* – which Fernando recommended to me – talks about the loss of materiality, of matter, in architecture. This brief work is a profound treatise on the pre-eminence of the vertical and hierarchical – could we say patriarchal? – a vision that has been dominant for the last few centuries. This Cartesian vision, far from the Spinozist treatises, discards a tactile, organic approach to spaces and the world. We have abandoned an existential vision, a phenomenological approach to focus on strategies of scopic advertising of instant persuasion. Buildings, Pallasmaa writes, "have become image-products detached from existential depth and sincerity" (2021, p. 28), losing the Bejaminian "aura" (Benjamin, 2003), becoming flat, immaterial and unreal decorations.

Tzvetan Todorov (2000) differentiates between two types of memory: literal and exemplary. While literal memory sees the past as singular and non-repeatable, Todorov suggests exemplary memory as a form of memory that involves retrieving the past and transforming it into a guiding principle for present actions. Memory, which filters and emerges in the present from the past, puts in tension the debate on the future and warns us of decisions for the future. Like the beams of previous centuries that express their reaction to the current cold or heat, like those apparently fragile ropes that resist the passing of the years and coexist with new ones, the memory of the past is a symbol of the present.

In that former bathroom, amid the amalgam of rubble, smells and textures, the materials expressed their history, their age, their origins and their use. Like our body and the wrinkles that run like paths across our worn skin, adhere to our bones with arthritis, linger and swirl in our scars, the remains, the debris spoke and made obvious what our society conceals: the fear of death, as Pallasmaa rightly points out. In this chapter, it is worth trying to recover the complex body of the world: its viscera, its origin, its age, that continuum of time that affects us and makes us re-think our connections, to go into the cracks in the wood, the consequences of a too warm summer or a harsh winter, to think of the cold, the warmth or the heat, the hardness or the softness, the slate or the marble. That slate, which today covers the floor of my bathroom and which everyone tells me "has stains" or "has imperfections", that marble of which I am told "some pieces are lighter", or "don't match".

Memory and trauma

Trauma is, by definition, unbearable and intolerable. The common ground of psychological trauma, according to the *Comprehensive Textbook of Psychiatry* (Sadock *et al.*, 2017) is the feeling of intense fear, fragility, loss of control and threat of annihilation. In this sense, trauma is extraordinary, not because it rarely occurs, but because it exceeds the normal capacity to adapt to life. The human being is left with a feeling without language, a pre-verbal feeling. The body becomes a symptom, reliving terror, rage or impotence, as well as triggering the impulse to fight or flee, to act or be paralysed, in ways and feelings that are impossible to understand and difficult to articulate. The body will probably "keep score" – like the title of Van der Kolk's work – for the rest of their life. Psychological trauma is thus an affliction defined by a lack of control over the situation, through an absolute lack of power over the surrounding circumstances.

At the moment of trauma, the victim is absolutely vulnerable, the power of a force that overwhelms them. When this force is natural, we speak of disasters. When the force is carried out by other human beings, we speak of atrocities. Traumatic events overwhelm the normal systems of care that provide people with feelings of control, bonding and meaning in life. The recognition of trauma and its treatment by medical and psychological institutions is fairly recent. The common response to atrocities is to make them disappear from our consciousness, at any cost – even our own emotional stability. Certain violations perpetrated in and by society are too terrible to utter aloud: that is the meaning of the word unpronounceable. Since the American Psychiatric Association accepted post-traumatic stress disorder (PTSD) in 1980, there has been acknowledgement and extensive study of the mechanisms through which human beings cope with the atrocity they have suffered or seen – denial, dissociation or repression, the intrusion into the person's psychic life and the marks it leaves on their body and relationships with others, preventing them from leading a happy life.

The effects on the fragility of the self

Qualities of the traumatic remembrance, of the traumatic memory, become difficult to describe in words or to integrate as part of the life story. The person, "pierced" by the unacceptable event they have experienced, is incapable of constructing a story, or telling it in an automatic (learnt) way, without being able to integrate it somatically into their personal narrative. Difficulty in processing information symbolically (verbally or otherwise) after trauma is a crucial element of PTSD. In fact, brain image research has shown low activity in Broca's area, which is responsible for the motor aspects of speech, and hyperactivity in the amygdala (fear, terror), hippocampus (memory) and occipital cortex (visual processing). What is basically altered is the autobiographical memory; the memory of the trauma is not constituted as a coherent story in which the aspects of the experience are fused into a narrative and integrated into the vital and intimate dimension of subjective time; rather, the traumatic recollections are constituted as separate fragments of consciousness that have not been integrated and remain disconnected from the overall story of the person's life.

Time standing still

In traumatic memory, the past becomes a past that does not pass. Trauma, also from a neurological point of view, is encapsulated in emotional memory, both individual and collective. The fragmentary and atemporal condition of trauma implies a lack of control on the part of the victim, which confers on traumatic memories an invasive and intrusive character that will continue to torture victims for an indefinite time, that will continue to be activated time and again, indefinitely. Atrocities, as history and psychology have taught us, refuse to be buried (Herman, 1992).

Overcoming trauma depends on the recognition and support of the society in which the traumatic event has occurred and the corresponding institutional and political bodies that assume the event as part of their mistakes. The study of trauma derived from war, for example, only becomes possible when there is a context that legitimises and listens to this pain.

In this way, and according to Herman, advances only appear when there is a social and legal movement strong enough to legitimise and welcome the alliance between researchers and patient–victims to counteract the common processes of silence and denial. Repression, dissociation, and denial are phenomena that occur in both individual and social consciousness (Herman, 1992).

Therefore, one of the most important elements in working with people who have suffered traumatic consequences of an event is the connection with the community and others. When trauma is the consequence of human action (as opposed to a natural event such as an earthquake or flood), the relationship with the other – the others as a community – is deeply damaged: a part of the primary ontological security is shattered and those relationships that were based on trust and affection may be irreparably affected for the rest of their lives. Symbolic restitution with and through the community is therefore of vital importance. Shame, guilt and the other emerge as key elements in this.

Processes of recovery of memory, whether oral, written or through various creations, have a therapeutic effect on the people who have lived through it, especially if those individuals find a listening community that can hear and validate their experiences.

Forgiveness: an essential element in trauma

To elaborate this part of the text, I have immersed myself in Jacques Derrida's work *Pardonner (Forgive)* (Derrida, 2012, p. 16f). Derrida begins his text by analysing the origins of the word and the action of forgiving in different languages. 'Forgiveness' is a noun. Its version in French, Italian, Portuguese, and Spanish comes from Latin and refers to 'gift', to 'donation', *per-donar*, implying a characteristic related to time and action, as in English, to *forgive*, and in German, *Verzeihung*.

There is particular interest in the analysis of the English language, in which Derrida notices the difference between *give* and *get* in the words *forgive* and *forget*, which means that, if we understand them as opposing words, to forgive is not to forget. Also interesting is the other German version, *entschuldigung*, or to de-blame. Thus, the meaning of forgiveness refers to an act – asking or giving – that links us to not forgetting and to guilt. The text also reminds us of the question of whether forgiveness refers to the individual or to the collective. Can there be collective forgiveness, which concerns a group of individuals? Who forgives, or who asks for forgiveness from whom? Who has the right or the power? And what is more important? "Who" or "what" to forgive or to ask for forgiveness: to forgive someone, or to forgive someone something? The who and what emerges again and again when we problematise the concept of forgiveness, as it speaks of the act and the perpetrator.

Between the individual and the collective

Derrida points out four ways of asking for forgiveness: "forgive me" (addressed to an individual subject), "forgive me" (addressed to several subjects), "forgive us" (addressed to an individual subject), "forgive us" (addressed to several subjects), where the singular and the plural are conjugated. These forms or conjugations link us to individual or collective responsibility, both to forgive and to be forgiven, and refer us to intimate individual and social action: is collective forgiveness possible? Is there a possibility of a forgiveness that is not singular, for a singular crime? These questions affect us in a clear and precise way and point to the heart of the traumatic process and its possibilities of recovery. Derrida points this out as one of the aporias – logical difficulties that are difficult to solve – of this question. Is forgiveness only possible face-to-face, without mediation, between the one who has committed the irreparable or irreversible evil and the one who has suffered it and is alone in being able to understand and accept or reject it? (Derrida, 2012, p. 16f). What offers greater personal and social restitution? To what extent is it legitimate? Do we have the right not to forgive? To what extent is an act forgivable, what extent is it not? Can there be forgiveness by a society, or can it only be done by the individuals concerned? Can an individual feel at peace because of the forgiveness that has been given by others? These are not easy answers, because they are not easy questions: they touch on the deepest vulnerability of the self and its relationship with others and the world.

In his work *Le Pardon*, Jankélévitch (Somme, 2011) points out three fundamental marks for forgiveness to be authentic: it must be a dated, concrete event; it is a gift, a grace from the offended to the offender; it involves a personal relationship. Also, Jankélévitch points out three forms of what he terms apocryphal forgiveness, which are not possible, of which we highlight two.

1. Temporal usury: in order to forgive, it is necessary to remember

One of the apocryphal forms of forgiveness that Jankélévitch points out is what he calls temporal usury, i.e. time. Duration – which heals, apparently – is, in Somme's words, a mediation of forgiveness in the form of forgetting, but the relation to time is not only forgetting; it is also memory. The development of time is thus equivocal, it attenuates pain and energy but has death as its horizon. Forgiveness, then, as temporal usury is a withering away, a decay, in the manner of senescence, a deadly or fatal process. That is why prescription or amnesty is not true forgiveness because forgetting makes existence disappear. And Somme points out that moral life should not be thought of in terms of continuity but in terms of perpetual rebirths. That is why "in order to forgive, it is necessary to remember" (Somme, 2011, p. 2).

2. The excuse

Another of the apocryphal forms of forgiveness would be the excuse, the understanding. Somme points out, interpreting Jankélévitch, that concealing the fault, evading it and understanding it, deprives forgiveness of its object and therefore its possibility. He thinks that if understanding can only be the way to forgive, it means, in a way, eliminating the wrongdoing, the evil, the sin in the offender, also implies an affective relationship. So, without denying the guilt of the act, it underlines the innocence of the intention. It separates the criminal from the crime and expects amendment. It removes, in a way, the reason for forgiveness and implies an affective relationship with the offender. The excuse is not forgiveness, the fact of being forgiven is inexcusable. Forgiveness does not ask one to diminish the offence in order for it to be forgiven, to be attenuated by the circumstances. Condemning the offence does not imply eliminating forgiveness.

Spanish film director Iciar Bollain's 2021 film *Maixabel*, which focuses on the relationship between a relative of a victim and the murderer, during the period when the Basque terrorist group ETA was killing politicians, state administration personnel and civilians, is an example of how not to conceal the fault, the horror or try to understand it. Featuring superb performances by Blanca Portillo and Luis Tosar, it is not about the executioner and the victim understanding each other, but about facing an act, probably unforgivable and imprescriptible. Looking each other in the eye, they recognise each other as human. There is no excuse, no understanding. No time can make them forget. Time in them, in both of them, has been frozen. Time does not pass; it is condemned to repetition. Until they meet. They meet even if they don't understand each other. But they recognise each other as human. The atrocity continues, without excuses, but Maixabell – the widow of the victim – manages to forgive, probably because she does not excuse either the other or the act, but she is capable of restarting a new time.

The imprescriptible, the inexpiable, the irreparable: the unforgivable

Jankélévitch, following Derrida, points out two axioms: the first is that forgiveness cannot be agreed if it has not been asked for. One cannot forgive someone who has not admitted their fault, who does not repent and who does not ask for forgiveness; the second is that when the crime is too serious, when it crosses the line of radical evil, when it becomes monstrous, forgiveness must remain among humans.

When forgiveness refers to crimes against humanity, they are imprescriptible and unforgivable. Is an act ethically prescriptible? Which acts are imprescriptible? Those committed against children, those committed against a people, those committed against women because they are women?

The poetic word

Abuses committed as referred above are extremely difficult to atone for, excusable and reparable. There is no place for collective forgiveness – because it is irresponsible – because there has been no place to legitimise the place of the victim, one by one, just as with their lives, destroyed one by one. There must be a place for the victim to stand as a person who can – or cannot – forgive. Society as a collective that embraces the victims in its community must also assume guilt, silence and responsibility. This fraternal word that Derrida and Jankélévitch point out is missing, this signifying voice that assumes responsibility and guilt, this voice that assumes the fault, the fault without reason, without understanding, without explanation, because it is not excusable. As Jankélévitch points out as a necessary axiom, forgiveness cannot be agreed upon if it has not been asked for. Because the victim is self-blamed, shame emerges as something unspeakable, and the community mercilessly turns its back on the victim. There is no fraternal word. The emptiness of impiety generates a pain that immobilises the subject from being able to go on living, from being able to trace their life. Faith in the other, communion with the other as an equal, as a neighbour, crumbles.

Demeter emerges, however, screaming and stops the buds of spring. We are faced with an evil that exceeds. There is no logical reason for forgiveness, no reason to forgive the unforgivable. The paradox remains: "Forgiveness is stronger than evil and evil is stronger than forgiveness" (Jankélévitch, 2015, p. 319). What to do?

Art as a possibility of forgiveness

Derrida's work includes several letters that open the possibility of communication or openness. And then, art appears. A young German, Wiard Raveling, writes to Jankélévitch:

> I didn't kill any Jews. That I was born German is not my fault, or my merit. Nobody asked me for permission. [. . .] If ever, Mr. Jankélévitch, you pass

> this way, call at our house and come in. You will be welcome. And feel safe. My parents will not be here. We won't talk to you about Hegel or Nietzsche or Jaspers or Heidegger or the rest of the Teutonic master philosophers. I will ask you about Descartes and Sartre. I love the music of Schubert and Schumann, but I will listen to the music of Chopin, or if you prefer Fauré and Debussy [. . .] It must be said: I admire and respect Rubinstein, I love Menuhin.
>
> *(Derrida, 2012, p. 47)*

If forgiveness does not happen, does not occur, is not given, is not asked for, is not offered, we are condemned to a past that does not cease, to a time that is detained and lacerating. A time that does not move, that consumes us in repeated pain, condemned to remember – over and over again – the ignominious.

Forgiveness, when it is given – let us remember the etymology related to the gift, *per-donar* – founds or allows a future, inaugurates a new time, a new life, and establishes another way of relating among humans. It is probably more related to silence than to words. While remorse is a soliloquy, forgiveness is a dialogue, it connects us to others. Remorse is closed, and forgiveness liberates. It is a secondary love, following Somme, it is the response to an offence. It is a counter-current love. But for it to happen, there must be community accompaniment, social and personal support, legitimisation, a symbolic embrace by the community.

This is what Wiard Raveling offers, without any justification whatsoever. For this reason, because Jankélévitch has found in him the fraternal, significant word, he answers Wiard Raveling as follows:

> Only you, you the first and no doubt the last, have found the necessary words [. . .] It is rare for generosity and spontaneity, for lively sensitivity to find its language in the words we use. And this is your case. This does not deceive. Thank you. [. . .]
>
> I won't go to see you in Germany. I won't go there. I'm too old to inaugurate a new era. [. . .] I've waited too long. But you, who are young, you, who don't have the same reasons as I do, you do not have the same insurmountable barriers to cross. For my part I will say to you, "When you come to Paris, like everyone else, knock on my door [. . .] we will play the piano."
>
> *(Derrida, 2012, p. 51)*

"It is rare for generosity and spontaneity, for lively sensitivity to find its language in the words we use," we remarked from the previous discourse. Perhaps art, the creative process – playing the piano together, without the need for words to get in the way – connects, beyond pain and words, the parts that seek and merge in aesthetic balance. That aesthetic balance that allows emotion, crying, mourning the loss of the one we were before the traumatic process, innocent and trusting. It offers a rebalance that allows us perhaps not to forgive, but to forgive ourselves, and for something to move in us, something that allows us to mobilise a mourning. Forgiveness, Derrida points out, does not come from understanding, but it generates understanding. Perhaps art, contemplating together the same work – Michelangelo's Pieta, where we recognise the immense pain for the young dead son; Medusa, petrified after having been raped and repudiated by the society that was supposed to protect her – moves us equally, makes us recognise ourselves as humans, in our humanity, makes us draw a line on a piece of paper, beyond words, that can point a way.

Matter as a cause and constituent of art: resonance and impact

How can art reconcile, how can it give form to a psychic gap without falsely closing it, how can it forgive and remember at the same time?

Aristotle pointed to the cause of substances – the formal, material, efficient and final cause – present in any work. In art, there has been much theorising about the history of the efficient cause – which passes from God to the human being – the final cause, discussing the purpose and object of the works, from purely aesthetic to instrumental purposes; likewise, the history of form and historical canons has been written about; but matter – that derives from the Latin *mater*, meaning mother, in relation to a raw substance – perhaps because it is considered the 'feminine' and mouldable element, has been overlooked and probably undervalued, misinterpreted and treated in a superficial way.

We are experiencing a crisis in the art system resulting from a concentration on the efficient cause on the one hand, and the formal cause on the other. However, in art therapy, matter convenes us with the world and informs us of our relationship with it, of our experience with the outside, with others and with ourselves. We take Bachelard as one of the few theorists who has devoted himself to developing a phenomenology of matter, a psychoanalysis at times of what matter says to us, as humans and what reverberates and resonates from it in us. For Bachelard, matter can be evaluated from two imaginative forces, in two senses – in the sense of deepening and in the sense of flight, both material and formal:

> Some find their flight in novelty; they rejoice in the picturesque, in variety [. . .] The imagination they awaken always has a springtime to describe. In nature, far from us, already living, they produce flowers [. . .] The other imaginative forces dig into the depths of being; they want to find in being, at the same time, the primitive and the eternal. In nature, inside and outside of us, they produce the seeds. Seeds where the form is subsumed in a substance, or the form is internal.
>
> *(Bachelard, 1942, p. 11)*

Within them, through the imagination of the materials, "they are dreamed substantially, intimately, setting aside the form, the perishable forms, the vain images, the becoming of surfaces. They have a weight, they are a heart" (p. 12). And he continues:

> Undoubtedly, there are works where the two imaginative forms cooperate. It is therefore impossible to separate them completely. The most dynamic dreaming (rêverie), the most metamorphic, the most entirely given over to forms, retains at least a ballast, a density, a slowness, a germination. In contrast, any poetic work that descends deep into the germ of being to find the solid constancy and the beautiful monotony of matter, any poetic work that draws its strength from the vigilant action of a substantial cause must, in the same way, flourish, organise itself. It must embrace [. . .] the exuberance of formal beauty.
>
> *(Bachelard, 1942, p. 12)*

For this reason, like Bachelard, and because we believe in the need to delve more deeply into the study of the constituent elements of the creative process on the basis of existentialist phenomenology, which obliges us to listen and listen to ourselves, matter is the key to our study and its evocations and has the capacity to incorporate our relationship with the world, to materialise it.

The artist as an aedo

The *aedos* (from the Greek ἀοιδός, *aoidós*, singer) were, in Ancient Greece, artists who sang epics collected from the population and set down in letters. They collected images – real or imagined – epic memories of loves and battles, of care and pain, of children, mothers, sagas and tales that were passed on by word of mouth, transformed into poems, tales and stories, as they wandered from village to village, from city to city. In the manner of the later medieval troubadours, they transformed real or imagined events, giving them aesthetic form through their works. With dispersed authorship, their contents came from the collective, diffused through time and space, from generation to generation. Only modern individuality has succeeded in stripping these works of the value of being the voice of groups and memory, of generations and cultures, in order to also construct a "property" of the common people. Homer was one of them. The function of art is to make the invisible visible, to give aesthetic form to what is given, to what is dispersed in the memory of people.

For some decades now, artists from different geographies have taken on the function of the aedo: they collect the pain and pathos of the collective, the open and painful gaps of war and violence, and give it form through matter or its immateriality.

The void: or how to sustain absence

Ausencias, Absences, is Gustavo Germano's masterpiece.[1] *Ausencias* represents the infinite and unfathomable emptiness of loss, in an infinite time and space. Through pairs of photographs, Germano shows time and space: memory of absence.

Gustavo Germano requests photographs from family albums of relatives of people who went missing during dictatorships – Argentinean, Brazilian, Uruguayan, Spanish. He invites the people present in the old photograph to take the photograph again, in the same place where it was taken, initially. However, this photograph now has an empty space of the absent person. This empty space of those whose fate or whereabouts nothing is known, who did not appear, never returned, who "were made to go missing".[2] Absence becomes present. The fact alone of returning to the place – a beach, the family home, the church where they got married, the gang picnic at a campsite at the weekend – adopting the poses we assumed in our youth decades ago, is an exercise in memory and mourning. Relatives and friends place the void in the space where a body is missing, in a time that has stopped.

The two photographs expose 20 years of absence and show the change in the space and time of the others. In front of these changing others, where time makes marks on the faces and colours the photographs, we see the motionless and inert stillness of a frozen image. As we pointed out in previous lines, the past becomes a past that does not pass.

Confronting the spectator with the pair of photographs brings back in an instant all the days, weeks, months, sunny afternoons and cold mornings without the loved one. Frozen. In an impossible mourning, without a body, the space is an unforgivable space, it is a cry of absence, and it is, at the same time, the sad look of those who were left, paralysed, by the absence. No one remains indifferent.

On the *Ausencias* website, "the missing ones" appear: in their absence over the years, but also, at last, in their names, their biography, their stubborn existence in the face of genocide. Matter, silver salts on photographic paper, emerges here as a search, precisely in its immateriality. The memory of what is gone remains frozen in the traumatic gaze of the others who perch on the frozen nothingness of memory.

The body as a vehicle for pain: hair as a symbol of identity

Art al Quadrat is an artistic collective that has been investigating identity, duality and separation for decades. The work *Yo soy. Memoria de las Rapadas* (I am. Memory of the shaven)[3] has become one of its major projects. During and after the Spanish Civil War, fascist troops carried out tasks of intimidation and public humiliation in cities, towns and villages. They took women, mostly wives, daughters or mothers of defenders of the republic or democrats and shaved their heads. Shaving the heads of human beings was and is a symbol of uniformity and usurpation of identity. In women, moreover, it is part of a visual identity that has been nurtured since childhood. It is not only a loss of identity, but also a loss of dignity. The women who were forcibly shaved, like animals, were paraded through the town in the streets and squares, to be the object of public gaze, victims of mockery, so that with a feeling of humiliation, guilt and shame, they would later confine themselves to their homes, and to serve as a warning and threat to the neighbours of the town who were watching.

Art al Quadrat, like Gustavo Germano, receives testimonies from women who were shaved, as well as from relatives who keep alive the memory of the humiliation of the act of public shaving and, in other cases, of the systematic rape and murder of women in the war and the post-war period.

Art al Quadrat launched an artistic event on November 5, 2017, in Sagunto, when the artists shaved each other's hair and performed the parade to which "las rapadas" were subjected, enacting with their bodies the memory and dignity of those women. In a step beyond the display and visibility of what has happened, they place their bodies and their hair, as a reversed act. They shave their own hair as a transgression, bringing to light a traumatic memory, on the

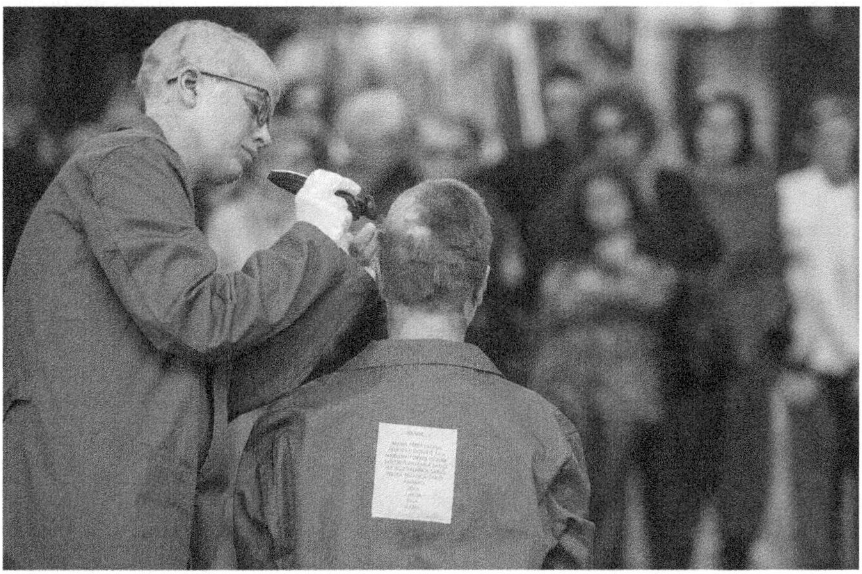

FIGURE 4.1 I am, *Memory of the Shaved*. Photo credit: Art al Quadrat.

public stage, in the agora, in the square. The hidden becomes public, it comes to light, and the hair becomes a human part that can unite: Art al Quadrat asks people to cut off a piece of their hair, to make a collective work with it. From that moment on, they collected testimonies from all over Spain and carried out public actions – wherever they were asked to – trying to stand up to humiliation and to make visible and give recognition to a wound that should never have been inflicted.

The hair emerges in its materiality, referring to a body, to life as well as to the rest, to the time during which the hair grows, to the hair, cut, separated from the body, as a trace of the identity lost as well as of the identity re-encountered.

Doris Salcedo: when the stone cries

Doris Salcedo has created *Palimsesto*,[4] a complex monumental work which, through the creation of a floor, allows drops of water to emerge, forming the names and surnames of people who have drowned in the Mediterranean Sea, trying to reach European shores. Starting from a dry floor of 400 square metres and apparently smooth to the eyes of the spectator, the names appear faintly and imperceptibly, because the typography inscribed on the floor is filled with water and allows the names to appear clearly and for a moment: Manal Eyoun, Abdulhamid Sheikh and so many others. The work consists of two overlapping cycles: the names of those who died during a migratory movement prior to 2010 appear in fine sand of contrasting colour embedded in the stone slabs; the names of those who died between 2011 and 2016 appear superimposed like drops of water that combine to form letters before filtering out again, in a constant cycle of inscription and erasure. Doris Salcedo manages to make the earth both weep and dry up in the aridity of nothingness.

Thus, drops of water continually emerge from the stony ground and slowly join to form the more than 200 names intermingled with the stories of these men and women (previously documented and researched by her team) who have drowned while trying to reach Europe in search of a better life. A solemn and silent work, a monument of mourning and pain. The stone exudes and emanates water that offers fluidity and drowns, escapes and dries. The smooth, impenetrable stone, ravaged by the memory of the nameless. Hard matter breathes out liquid matter, the water of the sea that drowns, the tear, also salty, that cries and takes shape, rewriting the forgotten names. As Bachelard points out, matter and form dig into the depths of being, they find both the primitive and the eternal in being.

"The whole idea of our society that you have to adjust and endure is unhealthy and creates more suffering. Our indifference is what creates suffering,"[5] says Doris Salcedo about her work.

Memory, matter, restoration: offer, sanctuary, relic, ritual

What does art determine, what does it discover, what does it summon from matter? It is the achievement of creation, as a state of exceptionality, that the experience of the visible and the tangible is made and remade before our eyes:

> aesthetic perception opens [. . .] a new spatiality; whereby the painting as a work of art is not in the space it inhabits as a physical thing and as a coloured canvas; whereby dance takes place in a space without objectives and without directions, being a suspension of our history; whereby the subject and its world in dance are no longer opposed, no longer separated, from each other; whereby, consequently, the parts of the body are no longer accentuated as in natural experience.
>
> *(Merleau-Ponty, 1975, p. 302)*

Creation, the creative process opens up to space, and in this opening up, it also discovers the irreducible. In the materials we will find gestalt and meaning, structure and imagination. But, beyond them, we will find our experience of them, our intercorporality through the visible and the tangible, confronted, accompanied by the experience of others. Those others who have caused harm or whom we have harmed.

The creative process works with openness without being a dual or hierarchical relationship. And the artwork, in its materiality, as a result of this, reopens in us the special moment where this relationship has been produced, a new spatiality that summons us as humans, in a movement inwards and outwards, a movement that Bachelard describes as vertical, but which could be a spiral. A spiral that runs through us in the creative process from the outside and inwards, placing us in relation with the outside and the others and, once realised, in its tangibility and contemplation from the outside, from the others, in the world and towards us. Memory and matter form a constituent part of art and its processes.

Through the metaphor of matter and the immaterial, of the evocation that summons, the three works we have described, *Absences*, *Memory of the Rapadas* and *Palimsesto* refer to concrete facts – people made to disappear by a regime of terror, women publicly humiliated, names of people forgotten and remembered only for a few seconds – which we recognise, through the matter of water, hair or absence, violence, pain and trauma. But, in a delicate and respectful way, it is shown to society: as an offering, a shrine, a relic or a ritual.

As in the mourning of the communities, society gathers itself – in *Palimsesto*, it was necessary to put on tights to cover one's feet, in front of sacred ground – and in silence, it walks carefully while watching the names appear, flood or disappear. Water that drowns and tears that weep. In *Absences*, in the form of photographic relics, we embrace and see the absent presence of those who have not been mourned, veiled or buried. In *Memoria de las Rapadas*, hair, an extension of the body, used as an ex-voto in many religions, is recovered in the community to honour those women who were dishonoured, and with the hair cut from the community, in a ritual of restitution, calm rises and breathing becomes rhythmic. Society, in silence, assumes its guilt, acknowledges and recognises the pain. And the aedo, the artist who shapes the collective memory reveals so that it never happens again. And the fraternal word, without needing to be pronounced, rises.

Perhaps, as Jankélévitch and Wiard Raveling pointed out, the absence of words and the aesthetic balance mobilise a frozen time that flows again – a sort of spiritual forgiveness – through the hug of the embracing community.

Perhaps these works help to inaugurate a new time, which remembers in order to forgive and establishes, as pointed out, another way of relating to one another, through silence, with the mediation of art.

Notes

1 To see the artwork: https://www.gustavogermano.com/portfolio/ausencias-argentina-2006/
2 A, unfortunately, very known sentence among perpetrators in Argentinian dictatorship, meaning the act of killing persons and make them disappear.
3 To see the work Yo soy. Memoria de las Rapadas: https://www.artalquadrat.net/portfolio/yosoy/
4 To see the Doris Salcedo's Palimsesto: https://youtu.be/L8vlSkmqtoE?si=EZyVQwi2JAsfyMVS
5 Interview with Salcedo.

References

Bachelard, G. (1942). *L'Eau et les rêves: essai sur l'imagination de la matière*. Paris: Librairie José Corti.
Benjamin, W. (2003). *La obra de arte en la época de su reproductibilidad técnica*. México: Itaca.
Derrida, J. (2012). *Pardonner. L'impardonnable et l'imprescriptible*. Paris: Éditions Galilée.
Herman, J.L. (1992). *Trauma and recovery*. New York: BasicBooks.
Jankélévitch, V. (1996). *L'Imprescriptible*. Paris: Seuil.
Jankélévitch, V. (2015). *L'Esprit de résistance*. Textes inédits 1943–1983. Paris: Albin Michel.
Merleau-Ponty. (1975). *Fenomenología de la Percepción*. Barcelona: Península.
Ong, W. (1982). *Orality and Literacy. The Technologizing of the Word*. London: Routledge.
Pallasmaa, J. (2021). *Los ojos de la piel*. Barcelona: Gustavo Gili.
Sadock, B.J., Ruiz, P. and Sadock, V.A. (2017). *Comprehensive Textbook of Psychiatry*. Philadelphia: Wolters Kluwer.

Somme, L.-T., Conference on Forgiveness with Vladimir Jankélévitch, at University of Geneva, 20 December 2011. Available at: https://jankelevitch.fr/IMG/pdf/jankelevitch-le-pardon.pdf (accessed 22 August 2022).
Todorov, T. (2000). *Los abusos de la memoria*. Barcelona: Paidós.
Vallejo, I. (2021). *El infinito en un junco*. Madrid: Siruela.
Van der Kolk, B. (2015). *The Body Keeps the Score: Brain, Mind, and Body in the Healing of Trauma*. London: Penguin.

5

VISUAL AUTOETHNOGRAPHY

A Transformative Practice of Remembering

Vera Heller

Abstract

This chapter describes arts-based, autoethnographic research that addresses the researcher's experience of growing up in Eastern Europe during the Cold War. This qualitative, first-person approach promotes the joint use of art and reflexivity in the exploration of a personal experience envisioned in relation to the cultural context in which it occurred (Patton, 2014). By establishing a link between the past and the present (Adams, Holman Jones & Ellis, 2015), visual autoethnography facilitates access to memory, both individual and collective. The first objective of this research is to explore the therapeutic impact of visual autoethnography and the second responds to the need to acquire a deeper understanding of the artistic component of art therapy. Indeed, the artistic dimension of the profession has received less attention from researchers in the field than its clinical counterpart (Kapitan, 2018; McNiff, 2013). Along the way, this objective has been attained through both my own creative process and through the learnings drawn from the work of three contemporary artists. The research project fostered a deeper knowledge of the therapeutic impact of visual autoethnography.

The results showed that the storied dimension of autoethnography serves to increase the coherence of the narrative identity while facilitating access to both individual and collective memory. On the other hand, the creative process involved in visual autoethnography gives access to tacit knowledge and original methods of enquiry, thus enriching the pool of artistic knowledge.

Keywords: autoethnography; arts-based research; narrative identity; artistic process; collage; memory

DOI: 10.4324/9781032663944-5

Abstract in French

Ce chapitre décrit une recherche autoethnographique basée sur l'art, qui aborde l'expérience de la chercheuse d'avoir grandi en Europe de l'Est pendant la Guerre Froide. Cette approche qualitative en première personne favorise l'utilisation conjointe de l'art et de la réflexivité dans l'exploration d'une expérience vécue, tout en la situant dans le contexte socio-culturel dans lequel elle a eu lieu (Patton, 2014). En faisant le lien entre le passé et le présent (Adams, Holman Jones & Ellis, 2015), l'autoethnographie visuelle donne accès à la fois à la mémoire individuelle et collective. Le premier objectif du projet est d'explorer l'impact thérapeutique de cette approche, alors que le deuxième visait vise à approfondir les connaissances sur la composante artistique de l'art-thérapie. En effet, la dimension artistique de la profession a reçu moins d'attention de la part des chercheurs et chercheuses que sa contrepartie clinique (Kapitan, 2018; McNiff, 2013). Ce deuxième objectif a été atteint d'un côté à travers le processus créateur de la chercheuse, et de l'autre, par le biais d'apprentissages tirés du travail de trois artistes contemporains. Les résultats obtenus ont démontré que le récit autoethnographique permet d'accroître la cohérence de l'identité narrative tout en facilitant l'accès à la mémoire. D'autre part, le processus créatif impliqué dans l'autoethnographie visuelle donne accès aux connaissances tacites et à des méthodes originales pour leur investigation, qui enrichissent le savoir artistique de la profession.

Introduction

This chapter discusses arts-based research titled *A visual autoethnography*. The project explores my experience of growing up in Eastern Europe during the Cold War through a series of collages, small memory-boxes, large format paintings and reflexive writing. My research objectives focus on a better understanding, firstly, of the therapeutic impact of visual autoethnography and, secondly, the contribution of creative work to enhancing knowledge.

Defined as a first-person inquiry, autoethnography connects lived experience to its cultural context (Patton, 2014). This approach to qualitative research is based on stories, which are described as "artistic and analytic demonstrations of how we come to know, name, and interpret personal and cultural experience" (Adams, Holman Jones & Ellis, 2015, p. 1). As my topic referred to a distant page of history, a variety of ethnographic documents consisting of photographs and written articles served to awaken memories of experiences and events while unveiling historical realities that had been falsified through propaganda during the communist dictatorship. Hence, they both facilitated and corrected my recollections, bringing about a belated understanding of my lived experience.

Through both concrete experimentation with art materials and constructing a narrative about my experience, the three-year autoethnographic process helped me to situate my narrative into its larger, collective context. My artistic work consisted of integrating photographic fragments into a series of collages and miniature theatres about both the past and the sudden occurrence of the war in Ukraine. The process of image-making has been healing in the sense that it enabled me to access tacit knowledge which had been obscured or forgotten. In addition, it allowed me to understand better the therapeutic function of the artistic component of art therapy. My new artistic knowledge has been enriched through the study of the works of Antoni Tàpies, Louise Bourgeois and Anselm Kieffer. The three artists succeeded in embodying personal lived experience into their art, thus offering a precious learning opportunity about the nature of the creative process and its narrative dimension.

The chapter will start with an overview of the research: I will situate it into the larger scope of a twofold project that extended the autoethnographic approach on a collective level and will briefly describe its second, group phase. The next sections will involve the exploration of the relationship between autoethnography and memory and the transformative capacities of both narrative and artistic creation. The significant learnings drawn from the practice of three contemporary artists will then be described as ways of enhancing artistic knowledge and the comprehension of the healing power of art. They will be followed by a description of the methodological bricolage that leads to the joint use of arts-based research and autoethnography. A few excerpts from my autoethnographic work will support the final discussion about its contribution to reconciling polarities, such as past and present, intellect and imagination, spontaneity and reflexivity. The chapter will highlight the therapeutic impact of this qualitative approach and its contribution to accessing artistic knowledge, thus underlining its compatibility with art therapy research, education and clinical work.

A visual autoethnography: an overview

The French writer Georges Perec (1989) prompts us to develop a questioning attitude towards life, which, according to him, may enable us to lay the foundations of "our own anthropology, one that will speak about us, seeking in whatever we have plundered for so long from others" (p. 9; Free translation). Perec's words reminded me of McNiff's (2013) call to access artistic knowledge and new methods of working, through our own artistic explorations. Indeed, as pointed out by Kapitan (2018), researchers in art therapy have mostly invested their efforts in the clinical dimension of the profession to the detriment of its artistic. Moreover, the psychoanalyst Didier Anzieu (1981) points out that, "the creative work represents the third most misunderstood form of psychic work" (p. 19; Free translation), the other two being the mourning and dreaming processes.

If, since 1981, much work has been accomplished in understanding the latter, artistic knowledge still needs to be developed. Several art therapists (Allen, 1995a; Kapitan & Newhouse, 2000; Moon, 1994; Sibbett, 2005; Politsky, 1995 all cited in Gray, 2011) have already offered examples of creative, autobiographical work in art therapy. Recently, López Fernández-Cao (January 2023) demonstrated that autoethnography can be used in teaching through the creation of artist's books as proof

> [. . .] of the power of the creative process to tell our stories, in an exercise of new lucidity and reconfiguration. They are, therefore, important examples for teaching reflection, since there is nothing like education to connect us with the other, make us responsible for him or her and reconfigure us as beings who accompany the story, the other's story.
>
> *(p. 189)*

As one's personal narrative is "at the same time the account of a community, of a society, of a nation, of an era" (Hillman, 2005, p. 91), autoethnography situates the researcher's individual story within its larger, collective context, thus offering another way of reaching other people who may identify or resonate with the experience (Adams, Holman Jones & Ellis, 2015; Patton, 2014). Although it was not my initial intention, my arts-based autoethnographic work integrated progressively both individual and collective perspectives.

I started my project at the onset of the Covid-19 pandemic, with the aim of revisiting my migratory journey through collage-making. However, I soon became aware that my images were evoking an earlier period in my life, that is, the experience of growing up in Romania during the Cold War. Thus, I was reminded that imagination is an autonomous entity, which obeys its own laws, linking images together according to a hidden, internal pattern (Bachelard, Levi-Strauss & Durand cited in Wunenburger, 2013; Ehrenzweig, 1967). McNiff (2013) acknowledges this reality as he points out that art "will always assert its unique nature through the spontaneous emergence of discovery, often contrary to plans and the most carefully developed strategies" (p. 7).

Following this realisation, I left aside my initial plan and decided to go with the flow. By allowing imagination to lead the process, I soon contacted an unexpected pool of memories about my experience of living behind the Iron Curtain. I started searching for documents and archive photographs that resonated with my own memories of that period and gathered personal travelling snapshots, photographs of previous artworks and sand play figurines. Using scissors, glue and paint, and a logbook for reflexive writing, I slowly crafted my personal anthropology. At first, I fragmented parts of these raw materials and then I incorporated them into new images consisting of a series of collages and miniature theatres. The wealth of available documents on the internet made me acutely aware that millions of Eastern European people witnessed the same historical events as I did. My autoethnographic process has progressively deepened, unveiling historical realities that had been obscured by propaganda at the time I was growing up.

The successive confinements and the wearing of masks that became the symbols of the Covid-19 pandemic somehow evoked in my imagination the reality of being silenced and locked up behind the Iron Curtain during the communist dictatorship. Working in a sustained manner on my visual narrative during Covid-19 highlighted the role of art-making in helping me escape the reality of successive confinements. In my artworks, the Covid symbols became metaphors for the impossibility of expressing one's feelings or going to see what life looked like on the other side of the Iron Curtain. The scarcity of outer space prompted me to enlarge my inner world through imagination, thus enabling me to experience the capacity of creativity to express human freedom (Durand, cited in Wunenburger, 2013), even in painful or dramatic circumstances. In one of his literary reviews, Herman Hesse (cited in Bachelard, 2014) tells the story of a prisoner

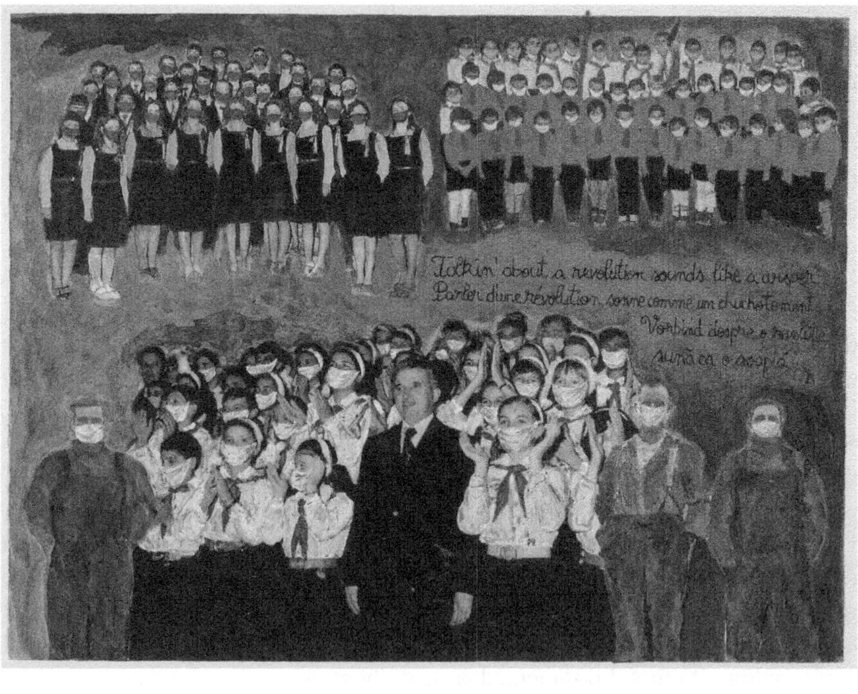
Talkin' about a revolution sounds like a
Parler d'une révolution sonne comme un chuchotement
sună ca o șoaptă

FIGURE 5.1 *Speaking Tongues* (2020), 14″ × 18″, mixed media on paper. Credit: Vera Heller.

who paints on the wall of his cell a miniature train entering a tunnel, imagining that he escapes his jailers by disappearing into its darkness.

> How many times poet-painters, in their prisons, have broken through walls, by way of a tunnel? How many times, as they painted their dreams, they have escaped through a crack in the wall! If need be, mere absurdity can be a source of freedom.
>
> *(p. 168)*

When the war in Ukraine burst into the news, I was already well advanced in my process of exploring an almost forgotten page of history. The war brought it again to the forefront, thus highlighting the relevance of my inquiry. The new 'Cold War perfume' evoked by the media was now being spread over the world. Its two greatest powers were once again crossing swords. I staged my perception in a series of miniature theatres titled *Pandora's Boxes.*

The inquiry into my own experience represents the first phase of a twofold research project. Titled *My Life, an Artist's Book*, the second phase is envisioned as a means of validating the results of the first one through the exploration of autoethnography with a group of seven participants of various cultural origins. Consisting of individual interviews followed by 12 art therapy workshops, the second part of the project considers the participants' migratory episode as one of the chapters of a symbolic artist's book that covers their entire life story.

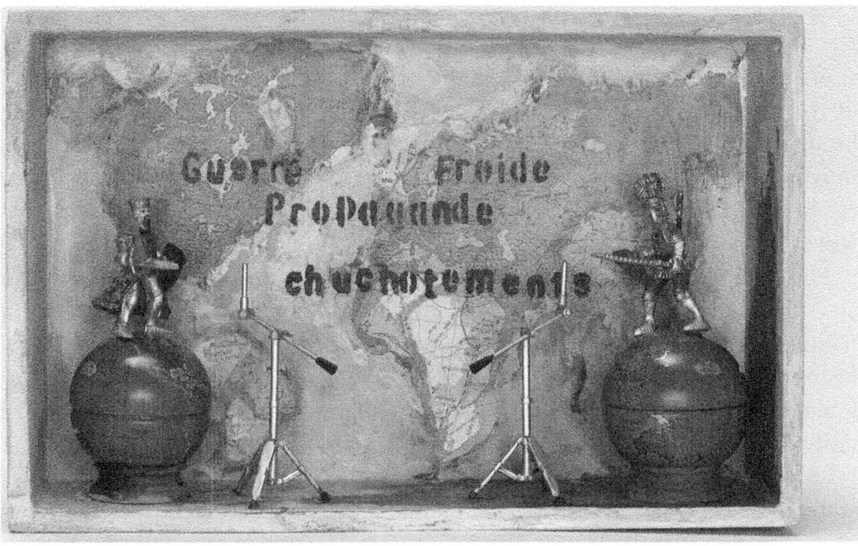

FIGURE 5.2 *Pandora's Box: New Crusade* (2022), 6″ × 9″, mixed media and wooden box. Credit: Vera Heller.

The experience of the four participants who came from Eastern Europe proved to be both similar to, and different from, mine.

Remembering

> Remembering is a commemoration, a ritual reminder that our lives address to the images in the background of the soul. By remembering, we provide a sort of commemorative legend, a founding image for our current existence.
>
> *(Hillman, 2005, p. 84; Free translation)*

For Friederich Hegel (cited in Dreifuss-Kattan, 2016), "to remember is to transform or to interiorize", and "to re-member is a way of overcoming the past by integrating one's memories into the Self" (p. 33). I have experienced both statements through my own creative process, whose internal logic brought me to remember an experience that I have never shared. Like many other stories that can hardly be voiced because of a lack of words, mine would have disappeared into the darkness of my memory if I hadn't started this process. The difficulty of defining in words traumatic experiences is also mentioned by Schwab (2010; cited in Pol, 2018, p. 88):

> How can one write a narrative about (something that) cannot be spoken and yet avoid creating a crypt in language? This question marks the distinction between a narrative that merely informs and one that performs an act of witnessing.

My own testimony is made of images. For Bergson (1959, cited in Touboul, 2016), they represent the only way of grasping the past. My image-making brought me to reflect upon the process of transformation of concrete memories into an imaginative narrative that I can own. It felt as if a missing piece of a confusing puzzle was progressively falling back into place. Later came the words.

Photographs represent an evocative form of documentation when used in autoethnographic work (López Fernández-Cao, January 2023). Using them facilitated the emergence of my memories; as stated by Hirsch (March 1, 2008), historical photographs from a traumatic past authenticate its existence. I integrated fragments of photographs into my collages, and I painted them over to unify the whole. The art historian Corina Ilea (2017) points out that Romanian history involves a belated understanding of the trauma from those who have suffered it, as the living reality was continuously being obscured through propaganda. Because of the "[. . .] continuously missed encounter with the historical event that produced it, not completely recalled, not completely possessed, and ultimately, not completely reliable" (p. 236), people have been left with nothing to remember. Given these realities, I believe that the generation who grew up during the communist dictatorship and the generation that followed but had no direct experience of it, both bear the trauma in similar ways. In Romania – and possibly in other countries that used to belong to the ancient Eastern Bloc – Hirsch's (October 1, 2015) notion of post- history that consists of the intergenerational transmission of trauma, may apply to both the generation who experienced it and the next ones. Nonetheless, art allows artists to grasp the fleeting memories of a confusing past through acts of imagination and fictionalisation, thus saving them from complete oblivion, and even more so when these artists happen to be immigrants (Ilea, 2017).

The transformative power of stories

> A story is the crossover point between oneself and the others: the narrator's story is a unique individual version of everybody's experience.
>
> *(Mitchell, 2012, p. 53)*

Although the terms story and narrative can be used in an interchangeable manner (Kim, 2016), the autoethnographic approach privileges the first. The postmodern dimension of autoethnography emphasises the limits of scientific knowledge regarding identities, lives and relationships, encouraging researchers to refer to their own experiences. Crafting stories through various forms of artistic and written expression favours reflexive self-exploration (Adams, Holman Jones & Ellis, 2015). They are works in progress with multiple versions of oneself, which is articulated around autobiographical remembering (Brockmeer, 2015). Sharing them with others is a type of social practice that infuses people's lives with new meanings while enhancing communication and reliance (Adams, Holman Jones & Ellis, 2015; Brockmeer, 2015).

As they tell their stories, humans are brought to reflect upon past events through the lens of the present. Reviewing one's life experiences contributes to bringing some order into the apparent chaos of life and, therefore, reconfiguring their narrative identity (Kim, 2016; McAdams, 2019; Ricœur, 1990). Life stories "mobilise aspects that help us to look at ourselves from other perspectives beyond those where we have been located or have unconsciously located ourselves" (López Fernández-Cao, January 2023, p. 191). For Ricœur (1983–1985, cited in De Ryckel & Delvigne, 2010), recounting them represents the best way of answering the question *Who am I?* If the answer to this question is fundamental for all human beings, it is even more so for people whose experience of displacement urges them to make sense of their living in more than one symbolic universe and not feeling at home in any of them (Brockmeer, 2015). According to Ritivoi (2002, cited in Brockmeer 2015), the migratory experience heightens self-reflexivity. Going through radical changes elicits a particular narrative attitude that contributes to people's efforts to make sense of the uncertainty. During the group phase of this project, I noticed the expression of the narrative attitude mentioned by Ritivoi (2002) through the participants' deep investment in crafting and sharing their original autoethnographies. Although each participant approached her or his own process in a unique way, all of them experienced the joint powers of storytelling and art as highly transformative. They all felt that the autoethnographic approach contributed to reshaping their narrative identities.

The transformative power of art

A sabbatical year offered a precious time that enabled me to explore the therapeutic benefits of a sustained artistic process. Having time supported me in the transformation of memories which had been threaded with trauma into a more integrated "memorial" (Dreifuss-Kattan, 2016) of my experience, and in the embodiment of tacit knowledge into visible forms (Barone & Eisener, 2012).

My artistic work has an intuitive, spontaneous dimension. Sometimes, it connected me with memories of concrete events, while other times it led me to associate chaotic mnemonic fragments in surprising combinations. As mentioned earlier, the physical work consisted of tearing raw materials into pieces, which I then reconfigured and unified by painting over the new images. The entire process recalled the continuous deconstruction and reconstruction of my story. As she evokes the making of her autoethnography, Goode (2023) compares her texts to the process of (re)assembling fragments through acts of memory or (re)membering. For her, the action of tearing and refashioning recalls the course of human life, which consists of a "series of fragments dispersed along the way and which we are constantly collecting up in order to reassemble them into some kind of container in which to hold ourselves intact" (p. 17). She compares her autoethnographic process to the Japanese art of kintsugi, a technique that consists of repairing a broken pot by assembling its fragments with a powdered gold mixture that leaves the cracks visible as a record of life. For me, Goode's (2023) comparison between the making of an autoethnography and the way humans construct their life stories evokes Ehrenzweig's (1967) theory regarding the function of the artistic process. According to Ehrenzweig, creative work consists of integrating dispersed fragments of experiences into a new whole, which involves artistic and psychic processes that go on in parallel. Although he does not mention the technique of collage, his description suggests parallel processes.

> Collage mirrors our contemporary realities by holding together several fragments that used to exist separately, thus permitting the co-existence of various perspectives into a coherent visual whole, a multifaceted image.
>
> *(Heller, 2007, p. 309)*

Three artists' work, a source of learning

Although none of the three artists discussed in this section envisioned their work as autoethnographic, it nonetheless recalls the approach of arts-based autoethnography, demonstrating, as pointed out by Touboul (2016), that art involves the cooperation between imagination and memory. Antony Tàpies, Louise Bourgeois and Anselm Kieffer's lifelong processes highlight the constant back-and-forth movement between imagination and deep reflexivity as well as various ways of integrating existential experience into art.

Tàpies and Bourgeois' prolific writings describe how they succeeded in transforming their suffering into artistic vocations. Their deep reflexivity contrasts with the spontaneity of their concrete art-making. As health ailments, fascism and the civil war overwhelmed Tàpies, making his life increasingly intolerable, he clung to art as his last resort. He later identified these difficulties as representing the roots of his artistic vocation and dedicated his work to healing others. He envisioned his artworks as power objects imbued with a curative function (Ishagpour, 2006). As for Louise Bourgeois, she used her art to manage chronic

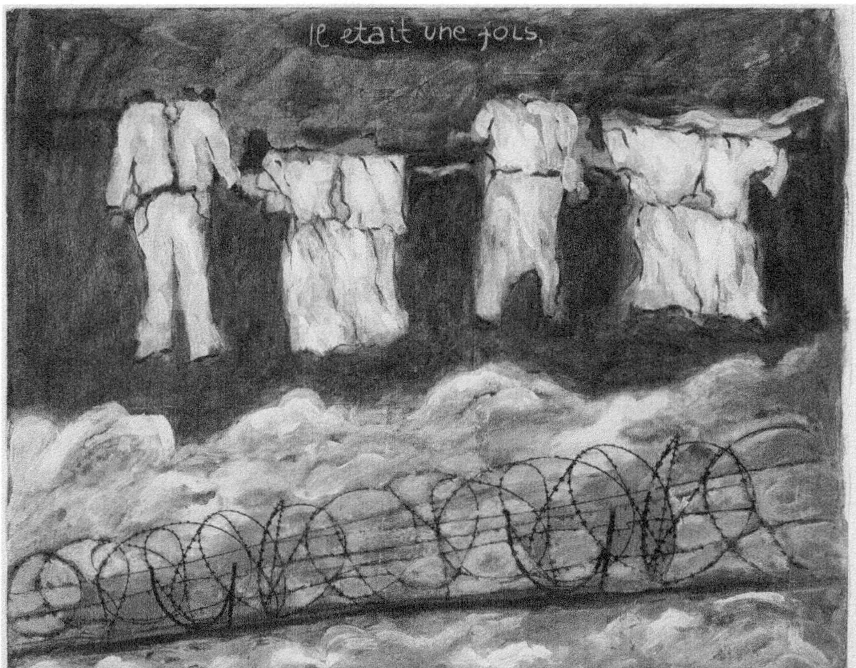

FIGURE 5.3. *Memorial* (2020), 14" × 18", mixed media on paper. Credit: Vera Heller.

depression and anxiety. She states that art helped her to become self-reflective instead of self-absorbed, and to deal with her anxiety in a more conscious manner. For her, art represented the highest form of existence, a way of "repairing" her inner world (Kuspit, 2012). Born at the end of the Second World War, Anselm Kiefer's whole body of work draws its existential depth from the destruction of his home by a bomb at the very start of his life.

The works of these three artists evoke memories in different ways. For example, one of Tàpies's techniques consists of imprinting the mark of an object into the thickness of the paste by direct application, with the intention of metaphorically restoring his memories about absent people or things (Frechuret, 1999). At the age of 86, Louise Bourgeois started to create a series of fabric heads. They represent her attempts to restore her childhood memories when she was repairing damaged tapestries in her parents' atelier in Paris (Rugoff, 2022). Anselm Kiefer reframes the notion of memory through the method of describing aspects of the past in new ways. One of his installations features an ensemble of shelves filled with gigantic books made from lead and steel, representing resistance against the flux of time (Brockmeer, 2015). Kiefer's paintings focus on the collective memory of the Holocaust and on the human suffering it entailed and tell stories about the hidden aspects of history (Arasse, 2001).

Long before my father told me his survivor's story, I felt deeply moved by movies and artworks such as Kieffer's that were evoking people's suffering during the Holocaust. According to Hirsch (1 March 2008), whether the transmission has taken place on an unconscious or an emotional level, the trauma becomes part of the next generation's own memories. Kieffer's work gave me the courage to confront them and bring into being my own memorial.

The joint powers of art and narrative: a methodological bricolage

The methodology of arts-based research and that of autoethnography present many similarities, of which the back-and-forth movement between imaginative processes and reflexivity is the most salient. Both methods integrate these polarities into a larger whole, which incorporates them in an organic manner. The two methods enjoy a reciprocal partnership that enhances the possibilities of both fields, their blending heightening reflexivity and highlighting the specificities of the creative process (Bartleet, 2022). Their compatibility facilitates a methodological bricolage that includes both (Bakan, 2014; Denzin & Lincoln, 2011; Kincheloe, 2001, all cited in Michaud, 2020). As autoethnography can be articulated visually, the field of creative arts may benefit from its contributions to enhance its own modes of inquiry. A collective of researchers in arts therapies calls the blending of the two methods arts-based research through autoethnography. Advocating for the use of art at most stages of the inquiry, they define their approach as an aesthetic way of knowing that remains as close as possible to the therapeutic experience (Green, Levey, Evans & Lawson, 2021). My own methodological bricolage has enabled me to access memories according to an aesthetic mode.

The first-person approach of autoethnography recalls the heuristic mode of knowing. In both approaches, the new knowledge is generated from the researcher's inner experience. Both incorporate creative processes in their methodologies. Like autoethnography, heuristic research can embody the researcher's experience into artistic or poetic depictions (Moustakas, 1990). However, as mentioned by Patton (2014), autoethnography aims to establish a relationship between the researcher's experience and its cultural context, an objective that does not always apply to heuristic research.

A few excerpts from *A visual autoethnography*

"An iron curtain has fallen across the continent," said Winston Churchill in 1946. I was born in one of these countries that was cut off from the rest of the world by an iron curtain, which remained in place during the following five decades.

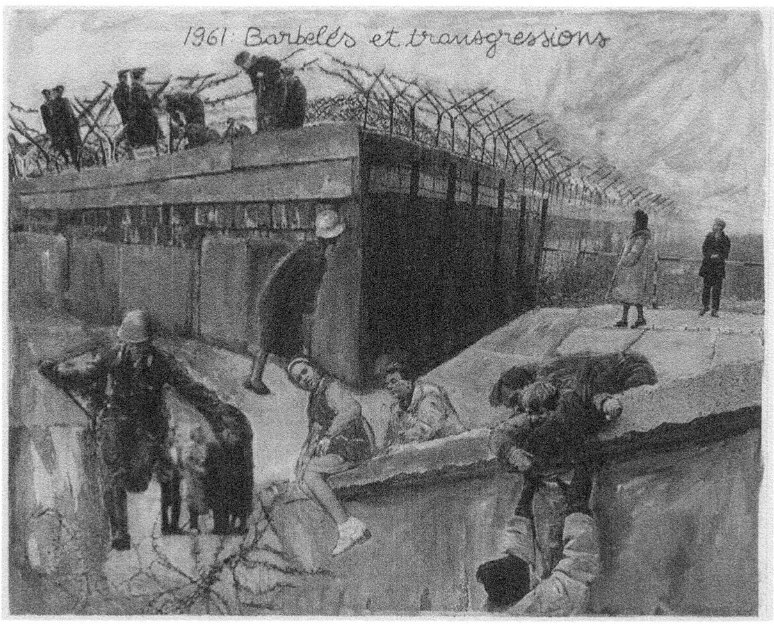

FIGURE 5.4 *No Man's Land* (2020), 14″ × 18″, mixed media on paper. Credit: Vera Heller.

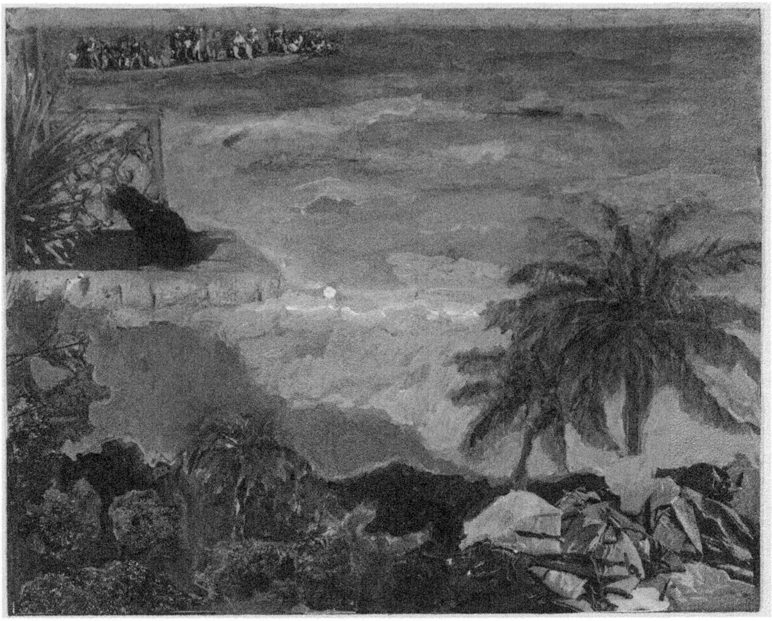

FIGURE 5.5 *The Boat* (2020), 14″ × 18″, mixed media on paper. Credit: Vera Heller.

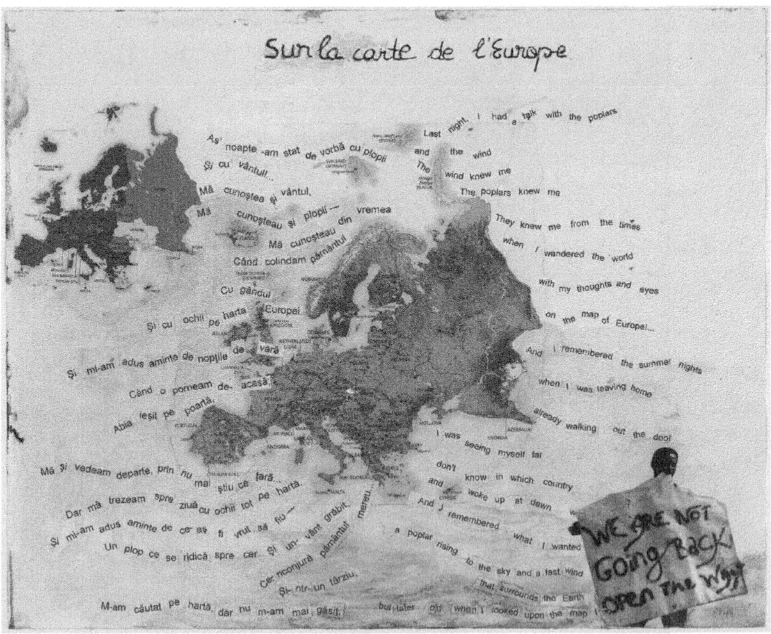

FIGURE 5.6 *On the Map of Europe* (2020), 14″ × 18″, mixed media on paper. Credit: Vera Heller.

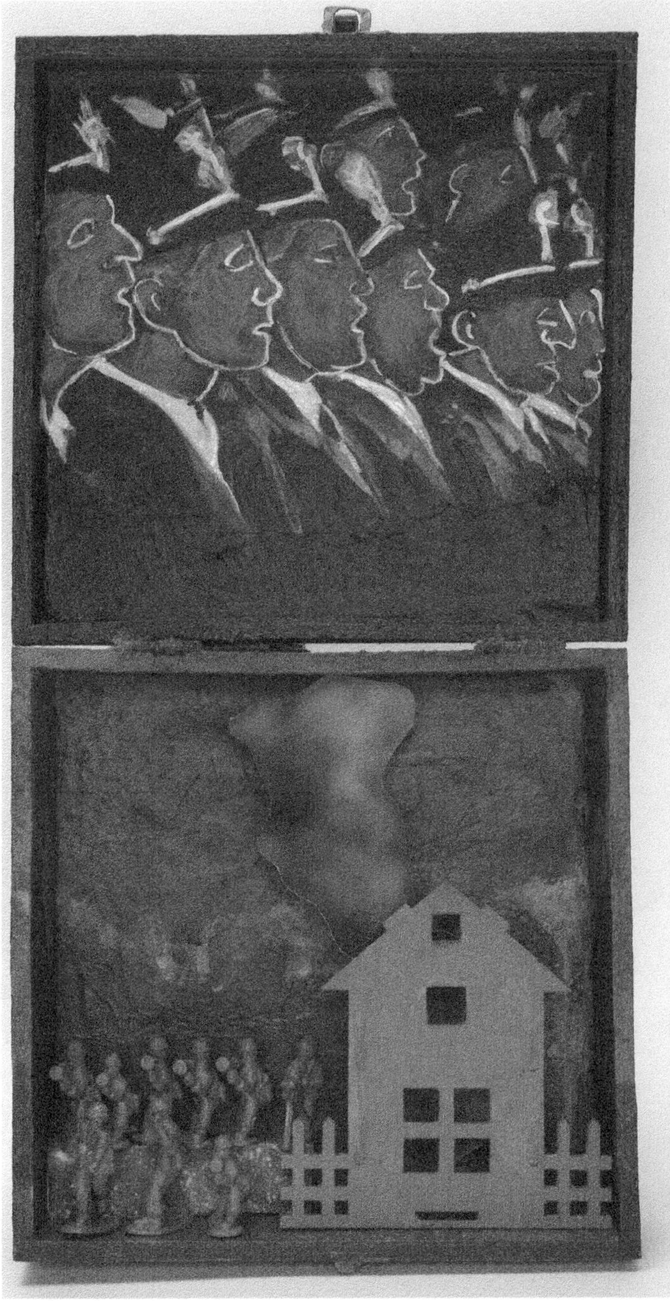

FIGURE 5.7 *Pandora's Box: A War* (2021), 9″ × 12″, mixed media, wooden box, sand play figurines. Credit: Vera Heller.

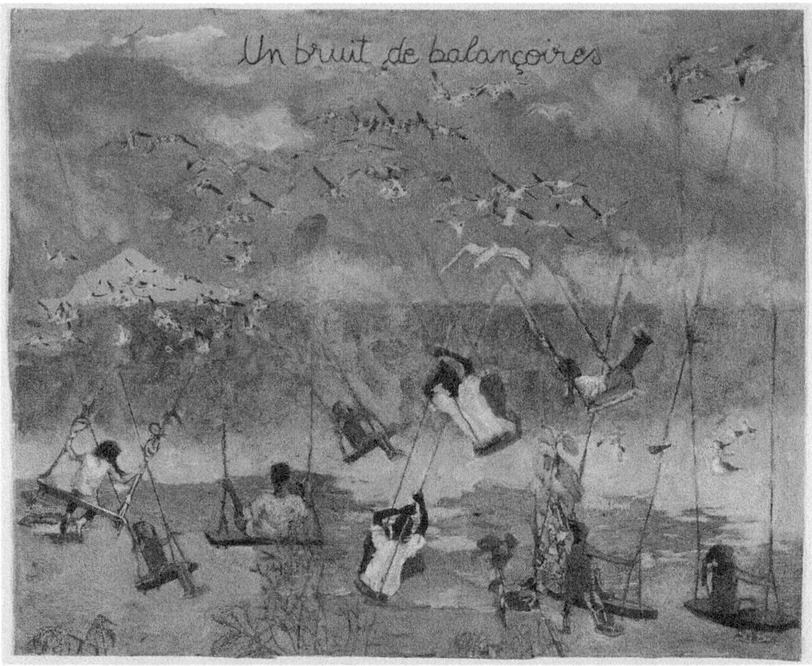

FIGURE 5.8 *I Used to Associate the Black Sea with Peace and Freedom* (2020), 14″ × 18″, mixed media on paper. Credit: Vera Heller.

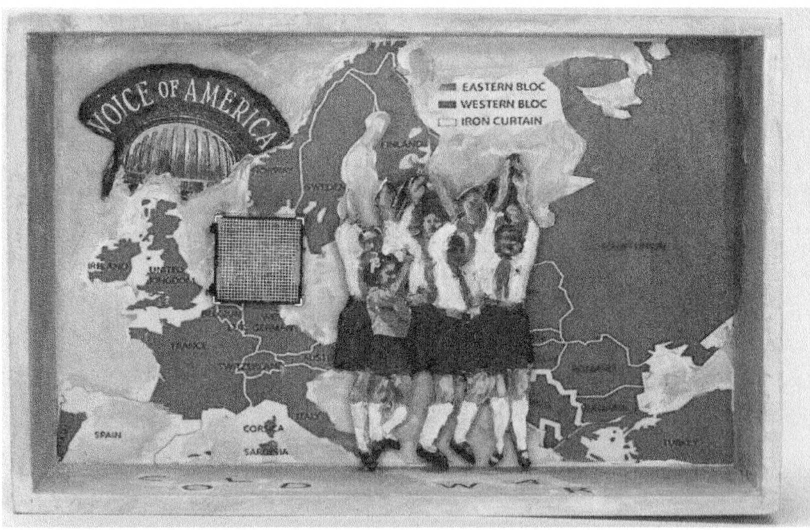

FIGURE 5.9 *Pandora's Box: Voice of America* (2022), 6″ × 9″, mixed media and wooden box. Credit: Vera Heller.

To maintain this separation, everywhere before us, lines of barbed wire were erected, and the no-man's land between guarded by soldiers armed to the teeth.

They were not that different from the ones that are being erected today in front of migrants.

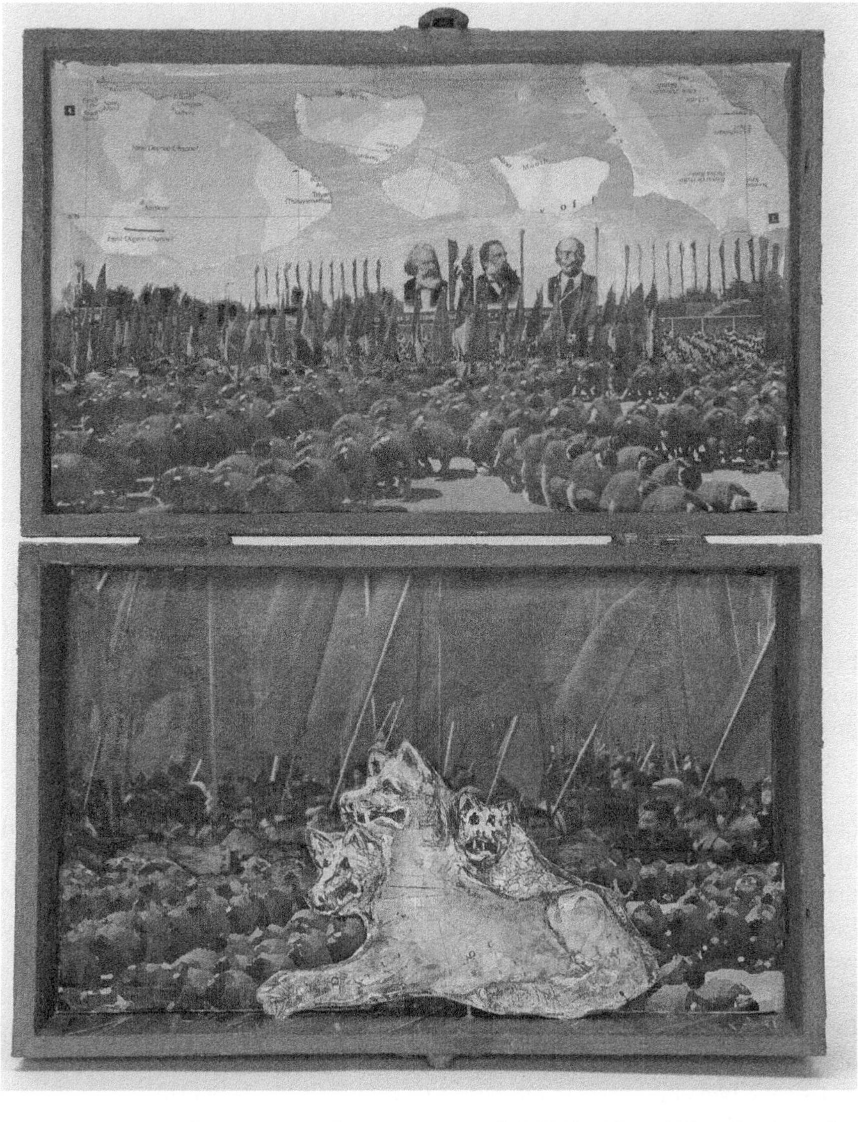

FIGURE 5.10. *Pandora's Box: The International* (2022), 9″ × 12″, mixed media, wooden box. Credit: Vera Heller.

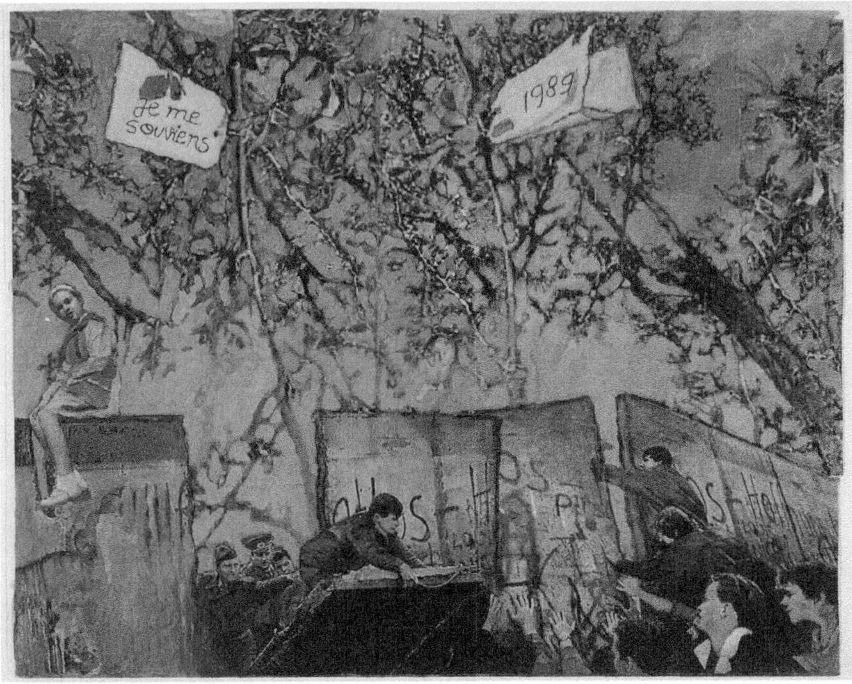

FIGURE 5.11. *The Wall* (2020), 14″ × 18″, mixed media on paper. Credit: Vera Heller.

During our geography lessons, we were learning how to draw the map of Europe. We were drawing borders, cities, mountains, valleys and rivers, without knowing that the continent was divided like a pie, between two great appetites, that it was cut in two pieces by the knife of history.

History repeats itself in new forms, and one day the war has started again.

Today, as in the past, giving free rein to one's words is not without consequences. The presidents arriving from the other side of the Iron Curtain used to smile and wave their hands, implying that everything was fine. I remember that people were secretly listening in to forbidden radio stations like Radio Free Europe and Voice of America. Their fictions were just the opposite of ours, they were about the world on the other side.

I remember the parades for the First of May and the lyrics of the mythic The International under the ever-present eye of Marx, Engels and Lenin. And one day, the wall that separated the two worlds has been torn down. Since then, other walls have been built; today, other Iron Curtains divide the world.

My creative process re-opened and progressed a story that would have otherwise remained fixed, one-dimensional and unsatisfactory. My relationship to this experience and memories continued to evolve to include new perceptions.

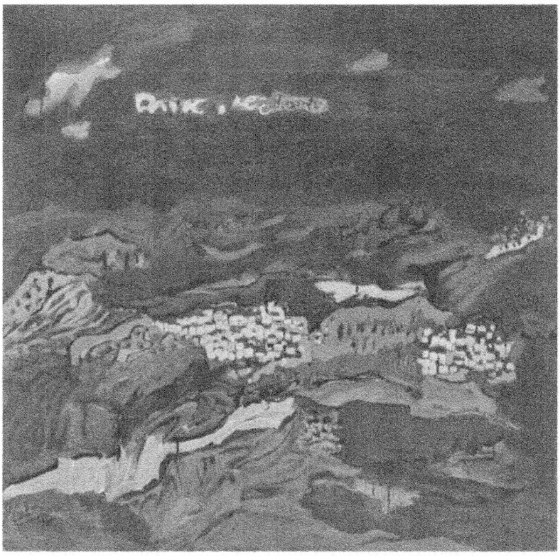

FIGURE 5.12 *This Story Goes Further, nb.1* (2023), 70 cm x 70 cm, acrylic on canvas. Credit: Vera Heller.

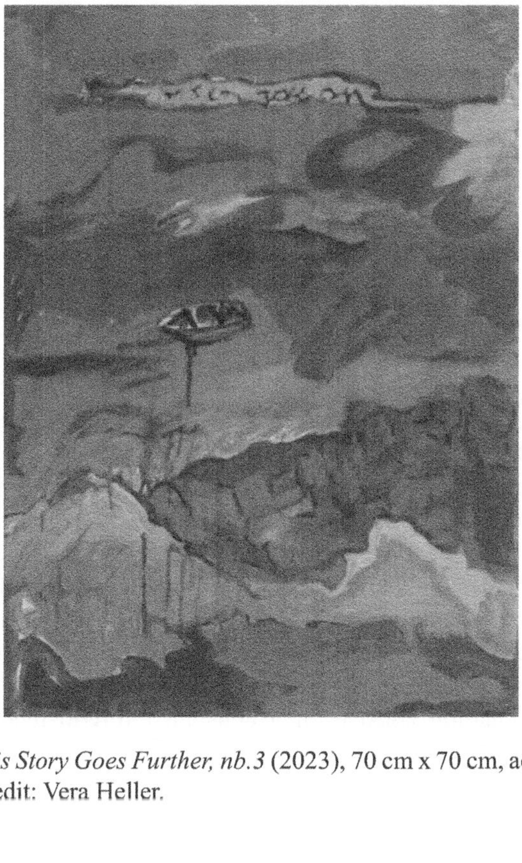

FIGURE 5.13 *This Story Goes Further, nb.3* (2023), 70 cm x 70 cm, acrylic on canvas. Credit: Vera Heller.

I recently returned to my country of origin to participate in an artists' camp. The colourful series of paintings I produced in this context evokes the joy of rediscovering places and people from new perspectives. The continuous process of de-forming and re-forming the story corroborates Ricœur's (1990) idea that our narrative identity changes as we reshape it along the way.

The healing power of imagination

This autoethnographic project started with my personal story and expanded gradually towards its collective, historical dimension. As pointed out by Gilbert Durand (cited in Wunenburger, 2013), our images are grafted onto an "anthropological trajectory" that begins at a neurobiological level and extends to the cultural level. Soon after I initiated my process, I realised it was taking me in another direction from the one I had originally planned. I was surprised to see that my actual images differed to a great extent from the ones I used to create before and that my memories that I used to take for granted became de-formed and re-formed into unexpected fictions. Jung pointed out that human existence is structured by imagination, and that our images are independent entities endowed with a life of their own. His ideas have been taken further by authors such as Gaston Bachelard, Henri Corbin, Gilbert Durand and Paul Ricœur, who, despite their differences, agreed nonetheless on the evidence that imagination has its own internal structuring laws, which are independent of our rational thinking and will (Wunenburger, 2013).

Corbin describes an "imaginal world", whose transcendent dimension is conferred by archetypes and myths, which are viewed by Bachelard as carriers of meaning from a universal direction to an individual one, and vice-versa. Similarly, Paul Ricœur and Gilbert Durand maintain that imagination is essentially based on myths, whose universal structure facilitates the staging and reconstruction of our narratives around the symbolic dimension of existence (Wunenburger, 2013). For my part, I spontaneously appealed to two of them, namely the myth of the hero, as represented by the character of Robinson Crusoe, and the figure of Cerberus, the scary guardian of the gate, as a metaphoric representation of the dictatorship and of the Iron Curtain.

According to Bachelard (cited in Wunenburger, 2013), human imagination owes its dynamism to a constant coming-and-going between two opposing poles: life and death, day and night, water and fire, active and passive. For him, the dialectic between opposites stands as the source of our ability to create. In an intuitive manner, I attempted to preserve the inherent tension between the two throughout my process, since I believe that the main function of any creative process consists of learning how to hold polarities together. In my understanding, individuation consists of a constant effort to reconcile opposites throughout one's life. Moreover, depth psychology parallels the development of an individual's creative work with its author's individuation process (Wunenburger, 2013).

I experienced the therapeutic impact of visual autoethnography through the creation of a series of collages and miniature theatres, a body of work that links my internal world to the external environment. Several times during the process I moved back-and-forth between the two, trying to bring into balance both my feelings and conscious perceptions. My perspective after having experienced such strong emotions during my work on the Holocaust prompted me then to create images that evoked happy moments. The back-and-forth movement between concrete artistic work and reflexivity contributed to my awareness that a longer-term creative process is a source of transformation and part of the individuation process.

Hillman's (2005) description of imaginative work as a careful collage of life fragments into a "narrative of the soul" drew my attention to the reparative function of collage. It contributed to my perceiving the action of assembling multiple pieces that evoke fragments of experience and integrating them through painting as a healing practice, which consists of distilling the raw matter of concrete events into a subtle matter. In my own process, the technique of collage fulfilled its therapeutic function by enabling me to integrate both my personal experience and the historical, collective events from which it has emerged. Indeed, as stated by Köhler (2012) "almost always political, collage is at once a technique and message" (p. 9). By its capacity to hold simultaneous processes of fragmentation and the reintegration of disparate pieces, the medium of collage mirrors one of the stylistic features of postmodernism (Heller, 2007). Kapitan and Newhouse (2000; cited in Gray, 2011) maintain that developing a postmodern vision in our profession has enormous implications for both education and clinical practice, as it allows the existence of a "highly relative, fluid reality that grows out of and matches the flux of the pluralistic, fragmenting culture we live in" (p. 11). For my part, the postmodern features of autoethnography enhanced my understanding of the social context, which is now organically integrated into my lived experience. We should perhaps consider the context of our preoccupations to a greater extent in art therapy since it fosters a better understanding of who we are.

Conclusion

This chapter has discussed an arts-based, autoethnographic research project, which explored my experience of growing up in an Eastern European country during the Cold War. As a distant page of history was being brought back to actuality by the war in Ukraine, the research proved its relevance by connecting the past to the present.

The overview of the project has been followed by a short discussion of the relationship between autoethnography and memory and described the transformative capacity of narrative and art. Their healing power has been revealed through my creative process, but also through the study of other artists' work. After offering a few excerpts of my autoethnographic research, the chapter has ended with some reflexive thoughts about the transformative function of imagination, which ensures the compatibility of this qualitative approach with art therapy research, education and clinical work.

The joint use of arts-based research and autoethnography enabled me to observe the contribution of the imagination in transforming memories of concrete historical events that used to be part of an untold story into a subjective narrative, which now belongs to my identity. The research contributed to heightening both my reflexivity and creativity while offering an imaginative answer to the question "who am I?" In addition to instilling a sense of inner coherence and meaning in my life, the autoethnographic approach helped me to define better my approach as an art therapy educator, artist and researcher.

These results answer the initial question of my enquiry, which consisted of exploring the therapeutic impact of visual autoethnography on the one hand, and the healing power of sustained creative work on the other. Above all, my learning from this long-term artistic and reflexive process concerns the autonomy of images and the capacity of imagination for self-structuring. I believe, if well understood and well used in the art-therapeutic process, these two characteristics of imagination can make significant contributions to healing memory.

References

Adams, T.E., Holman Jones, S. and Ellis, C. (2015). *Autoethnography: Understanding Qualitative Research*. New York: Oxford University Press.

Anzieu, D. (1981). *Le corps de l'œuvre*. Paris: Gallimard.

Arasse, D. (2001). *Anselm Kieffer*. New York: Abram Books.

Bachelard, G. (2014). *The Poetics of Space*. New York: Penguin.

Barone, T. and Eisener, E.W. (2012). *Arts Based Research*. Los Angeles: Sage.

Bartleet, B.-L. (2022). Artistic autoethnography: Exploring the interface between autoethnography and artistic research. In T.E. Adams, S. Holman Jones and C. Ellis (eds), *Handbook of Autoethnography*, 2nd edn. New York: Routledge.

Brockmeer, J. (2015). *Beyond the Archive: Memory, Narrative, and the Autobiographical Process*. Oxford: Oxford University Press.

De Ryckel, C. and Delvigne, F. (2010). La construction de l'identité par le récit. *Psychothérapies*, 30(4), 229–240. doi.org/10.3917/psys.104.0229

Dreifuss-Kattan, E. (2016). *Art and Mourning: The Role of Creativity in Healing Trauma and Loss*. London: Routledge.

Ehrenzweig, A. (1967). *The Hidden Order of Art: A Study in the Psychology of Artistic Imagination*. Los Angeles: University of California Press.

Frechuret, M. (1999). Antoni Tàpies, ou le pouvoir curatif du tableau talisman. In M. Frechuret, and T. Davila (eds), *L'art Médecine*. Paris: Réunion des musées nationaux.

Goode, J. (2023). Shoring up the fragments. In J. Goode, K. Lumsden and J. Bradford (eds), *Crafting autoethnography: Processes and practices of making self and culture*. London: Routledge.

Gray, B. (2011). Autoethnography and arts therapy: The arts meet healing. *ANZJAT-CATA*, 6(1), 67–80. https://www.anzacata.org/resources/Files/11_ANZJAT/ANZJAT-2011/8ANZJAT-2011-BG-A.pdf

Green, A., Levey, B. Evans, W. and Lawson, K. (2021). The arts of making sense in uncertain times: Arts-based research and autoethnography. In H. Kara and S.-M. Khoo (eds), *Qualitative and Digital Research in Times of Crisis: Methods, Reflexivity, and Ethics*. Bristol: Bristol University Press.

Heller, V. (2007). Exile, identity, and artistic creation: An arts-based phenomenological study with immigrant women. Doctoral dissertation, Lesley University. Available at: https://digitalcommons.lesley.edu/expressive_dissertations/33/

Hillman, J. (2005). *La fiction qui soigne*. Paris: Payot.

Hirsch, M. (2008). The generation of postmemory. *Poetics Today*, 29(1), 103–128. doi:10.1215/03335372-2007-019

Hirsch, M. (2015). Postmémoire: Témoigner. Entre histoire et mémoire. *Revue Pluridisciplinaire de la Fondation Auschwitz*, 118(114), 201–2013. https://doi.org/10.4000/temoigner.1274

Ilea, C. (2017). Migratory affiliations: Contemporary Romanian art. In M. Langford (ed.), *Narrative Unfoldings: National Art Histories in an Unfinished World*. Montreal and Kingston: McGill-Queen's University Press.

Ishagpour, Y. (2006). *Antoni Tàpies: Works, Writings, Interviews*. Barcelona: Polìgrafa.

Kapitan, L. (2018). *Introduction to Art Therapy Research* (2nd edn). New York: Routledge.

Kim, J.-H. (2016). *Understanding Narrative Inquiry*. Los Angeles: Sage.

Köhler, T. (2012). Manifesto collage: Collage in arts and sciences. In C. Zu Salm (ed.), *Manifesto Collage: Defining Collage in the Twenty-first Century*. Nürnberg: Moderne Kunst.

Kuspit, D. (2012). Louise Bourgeois in psychoanalysis with Henry Lowenfeld. In P. Larrat-Smith (ed.), *Louise Bourgeois: The Return of the Repressed*. London: Violette.

López Fernández-Cao, M. (2023). The artist's book as a form of autoethnography for the teaching profession: Reflections on the photographic act. In A. Bautista García-Vera (ed.), *Photographic Elicitation and Narration in Teachers Education and Development, Teacher Education, Learning Innovation and Accountability*, 179–197. Open Access. Berlin: Springer Nature. doi: 10.1007/978-3-031-20164-6_12

McNiff, S. (ed.). (2013). *Art as Research: Opportunities and Challenges*. Bristol: Intellect Ltd.

McAdams, D.P. (2019). First, we invented stories, then they changed us: The evolution of narrative identity. *Evolutionary Studies in Imaginative Culture*, 3(1), 1–18.

Michaud, A-M. (2020). *Auto ethnographie d'une artiste pédagogue*. Doctoral Dissertation, Laval University.

Mitchell, J. (2012). The sublime Jealousy of Louise Bourgeois. In P. Larrat-Smith (ed.), *Louise Bourgeois: The Return of the Repressed*. London: Violette.

Moustakas, C. (1990). *Heuristic Research: Design, Methodology, and Applications*. Newbury Park: Sage.

Patton, M. (2014). *Qualitative Research & Evaluation Methods: Integrating Theory and Practice* (4th edn). Los Angeles: Sage.

Perec, G. (1989). *L'infra-ordinaire*. Paris: Seuil.

Pol, A. (2018). Trauma y afectos: Las historias del cuerpo. Comment faire? Trauma, memoria, feminism, afectos. In M. López Fdz. Cao (ed.), *Arte, memoria y trauma: Aleteia, dar forma al dolor: Sobre Procesos, arte y memoria*. Madrid: Fundamentos.

Ricœur, P. (1990). *Soi-même comme un autre*. Paris: Seuil.

Rugoff, R. (2022). Mechanisms of ambiguity and sensation: The late fabric sculptures of Louise Bourgeois. In *Louise Bourgeois: The Woven Child*. Exhibition catalogue. London: Hayward Gallery.

Touboul, P. (2016). Ce que l'art fait à la mémoire: Le renouvellement éthique de l'appropriation du temps humain. *Nouvelle revue d'esthétique*, 2(18), 103–114. https://doi.org/10.3917/nre.018.0103

Wunenburger, J.J. (2013). *L'imaginaire* (2nd edn). Paris: Presses Universitaires de France.

6

WHEN I RULED THE WORLD

Adopted Children's Memories of Early Life Trauma Recalled in a Process of Meaning-making in Music Therapy

Joy Gravestock

Abstract

This chapter is a re-thinking of a paper given at the ECArTE 2022 conference. My paper included video extracts from sessions where adopted children were shown to have become more powerfully connected with pre-verbal memory that had been forgotten. In this chapter, I replace live video with written vignettes of casework. The casework illustrates how traumatic adoption-specific memory, once recalled, can be witnessed and held safely, leading to a reframing of narrative. Casework vignettes sit alongside my ontology, which theorises how I have come to understand how the music of adopted children expresses attachment communications at levels beneath conscious awareness within the dynamic intersubjective field (Robarts, 2014). Music therapy therefore becomes a language for affect-laden material, making unconscious relational experiences more conscious, more remembered. For an adopted child, the past can be then known in a new way, and new relational experiences within music therapy might be experienced. Ultimately, memory recovered can become memory repaired and children can take new relational repertoire into life beyond the therapy room.

Keywords: adoption, music therapy, traumatic memories, intersubjectivity, relational psychotherapy

Introduction

Adopted children's earliest lived experiences of loss remain embedded in their deepest cell memory. Infant adoptees absorb overwhelming sensations of abandonment, while not yet having acquired language to process and assimilate their

DOI: 10.4324/9781032663944-6

experience (Robarts, 2014). It is an adoptee's embodied state therefore that holds an internalised knowledge of early trauma. Unconscious pre-adoption experiences likely remain unknown to the adoptee but carry an instantly recognisable present feeling tone (Wilkinson, 2010). Memory governs problematic ways of being and behaving, evident in what Wilkinson describes as old material being manifest in the present, being alive still in the adoptee's internal world. It is this embodiment of adoption-specific trauma which often leads to referrals to music therapy with me.

Verrier (1993) describes the un-remembered loss adoptees carry in the body as an enduring emotional wound. This is encapsulated beautifully in the Welsh word *hiraeth* which means a homesickness tinged with grief, loss and a yearning for a place to which you cannot return. Adopted children long for that unknown place held in their embodied memory.

The pre-symbolic level at which music is experienced in the body then has a special role in working with recollections of memory in adoption work. Children can feel grounded in their own music-making, while processing and assimilating the impact of embodied memory because music offers, in Sutton's words, "experiences of our total selves as embodied in sound" (2002, p. 35). The intrinsic sensory modality and psychophysiological effect of spontaneous improvised music-making can help develop an adopted child's narrative of being (Trevarthern, 2009).

In music therapy sessions with many children over the past decade, I have been privileged to witness adoptees become powerfully connected with that which has been forgotten. When traumatic memory recalled in this way can be safely held and thought about it can lead to a reframing of narrative. The music of adopted children can express attachment communications at levels beneath conscious awareness within the dynamic intersubjective field (Robarts, 2014). The co-created music of music therapy therefore becomes a shared language for affect-laden material, making unconscious experience more conscious and more remembered.

This chapter will refer throughout to any members of an adoptee's "birth family" as the "first family" and refer to any members of their adopted family as the "second family." This is becoming the language of the adoption community and is the language most desired and chosen by adopted adults to speak of their experience.

Joe's memory

Joe was 11 years old and brought contemporary pop songs to his early music therapy sessions. Superficially, there was little that seemed remarkable in these songs and yet when he sang them within sessions, both the quality of his voice and the earnestness with which he sang them within sessions made them redolent with meaning. He began to favour singing "Viva La Vida" by Coldplay (one of many songs he potentially had access to in contemporary culture yet *this* one mattered) and repeatedly singing one verse. The repeated verse needed to be thought about differently in our therapeutic space, driven as it seemed to be by an unconscious choice. Joe's intense, urgent, agitated singing communicated his emotional distress. I had initially wondered if he brought pop songs as a defence to avoid entering into more exposing improvisations with me. However, in reflection within supervision, I began to understand that both the lyrics and the songs' musical structures were together providing an important vehicle of communication for Joe at a deep level.

Joe sang these words: "It was the wicked and wild wind, blew down the doors to let me in, shattered windows and the sound of drums, people couldn't believe what I'd become."

I met with Joe's social worker and together we began to search for any information about his early life experience. It transpired that the song appeared to contain an unconscious recognition of a pre-adoption narrative Joe could not consciously know he had. In fact, the verse he kept singing on repeat, as it were, directly described an extremely early pre-adoption experience of trauma within his first family. When Joe was 18 months old, his first dad had broken into his first mum's ground-floor flat, smashing the glass window of Joe's bedroom to do so. He had then taken Joe from home in a kidnap attempt. Soon after this Joe was removed from his first family and placed for adoption.

Joe had previously been missing, or choosing not to attend, his appointments with a local child and adolescent mental health services (CAMHS) team because he stated that he could not talk about adoption, as everyone around him seemed to want him to be able to do. However, attending music therapy, where he did not feel any pressure to speak, and rather seemed to be engaging in 'just singing stuff', enabled him to sing out an unconscious story that needed telling. Music provided some containment, self-soothing, and affect regulation for him where his unconscious early memory could emerge and be safely thought about with a witnessing music therapist who could also musically hold the shared experience. Music therapy seemed therefore to provide a necessary and modified response for Joe as he related musically from his deepest unconscious level. Memories and their expression were safely held within the musical relationship.

Memory

The theme of memory linking all of the chapters in this book is such an important one for me, working as I do within the field of adoption. Within adoption work, there is recognition that adoptees' earliest memories will be stored in the body. An adoptee who was removed at birth from their first family and placed quickly with an adoptive family will still have experienced huge trauma. The adoption community calls this the *specific* trauma of adoption. There is recognition that a baby/infant will not have a cognitive grasp of what is happening to them when they are separated from their mother but the experience will be held as a traumatic memory within the body. In my work, I recognise that such memory will be unconscious, but that music therapy can enable the expression of the unconscious and as such is well-placed to help with early trauma and embodied memory.

Memory was the theme of the conference from which all of the chapters in this book came, and the pre-conference information encouraged prospective presenters to think about memory from various points. Firstly, the pre-conference literature guided presenters to think about Plato's definition of memory as a recollection of an inherited knowledge. This connected immediately with my work (as described in the previous paragraph). Adoptees often refer to their "inheritance" within their birth family, which is often denied them (for example, adoptees lose their biological "inheritance" and often struggle in later life when asked to describe a medical family history). Adoptees retain some "inherited knowledge," however, which was passed from mother to infant even in the briefest moments together.

Plato also described anamnesis, which he defined as the calling to mind of a previous existence. This statement also resonated deeply with my work. It reminded me of the *hiraeth* experience I described earlier in this chapter. The vignette of Joe I described above shows Joe's recollection of the knowledge he had indeed inherited during his time living with his first family. It was a part of his existence and intrinsic to his fullest sense of self and identity. I think that Joe went through a process that we may describe as anamnesis as he called back into mind those earliest memories that continued to impact upon him.

Joe's music-making provided him with a way of gaining recollection of embodied memories, stored deep within his body. As he could find a way to recall his early experience he could then have a "re-remembering" of it. I spoke with an adopted child prior to writing this chapter about Plato's definitions and they said, "Yeah, that makes sense, cos doing music therapy helps bring back my forgettings." I cannot think of a better way of paraphrasing Plato!

Adopted children will almost certainly have needed to forget their trauma and necessarily employed mechanisms of repression, distortion of memory, denial and other defences to manage hugely difficult feelings. Music therapy can provide, possibly, something like Freud's notion of the "*après-coup*" (which I shall discuss further later in this chapter) to enable safe recall, sense-making and the creation of new experiences.

The conference (and subsequently this book) have described four ways in which the arts therapies can enable working with memory (ECArTE Call For

Abstracts, 2021), and below I have made these explicitly musical in the way they resonated for me:

a. The arts (music) have offered a means for memories to move away from literal narrative into symbolic and aesthetic forms. *Music provides aesthetic forms and structures which can express memory symbolically.*
b. The arts (music) invite a performative rendering of memory in all its forms. *Music therapy is less threatening to adoptees who cannot speak of their experience but can "perform" it to an audience of a therapeutic witness.*
c. The arts (music) can move memory away from sequential time, through the body, kindling a recollection of impressions. *The capacity to connect to songs and tunes can enable memory to emerge. The "old past" can be made anew in the here-and-now present.*
d. Memories are carried in musical notes. *They can be held and thought about in musical structures that provide safety and holding, so adoptees are not overwhelmed in recall.*

All of the above seems relevant to what I regularly see occurring in the music therapy room. I shall now go on to describe how I have theorised the way that playing music together in relationship can make a space for memory and also make reparation for traumatic early experiences.

Embodied memory: music-making and attunement possibilities

Stern's (1998) work on intersubjectivity introduces the concept of affect attunement occurring between mothers and their babies. This felt relational sense is totally lost for adoptees when the fundamental first relationship is totally denied to them. The impact of the loss of their first mother for any adopted child, even if they are only hours old when they are removed, can cause serious lifelong issues for an adoptee. Tiny infants absorb overwhelming sensations of abandonment, while not yet possessing the resources for language to process and assimilate this experience. Adoptees who were placed in their new families as babies, just days or weeks old, become those children and adults whom commonly I have heard describe feeling a "hole" inside themselves. This hole might function as a metaphorical description for adopted people; it is an attempt to describe impaired intersubjectivity which impacts negatively on their core of rhythmic and sympathetic impulses, as well as on developing brain connectivity, self-regulation and attachment capacity. In essence, the lived experience of "having a hole inside" stems from denied attunement experiences in the first family. This, in turn, inevitably impacts on attachment. What has been lost, though, is waiting to be recalled with the hope of this being possible and music therapy offering some degree of reparation and integration for the adoptee.

For adoptees, a music therapy relationship might provide a creative, safe space for a sense of attunement to be re-experienced. Attunement originates in non-verbal elements of communication and exists in the how and when of an interaction or exchange rather than its apparent content. It grows out of spontaneity, creativity and unpredictability in our work, which Stern (2004) calls sloppiness or intentional fuzziness. Working within a needs-led approach, utilising free improvisation, both the client's and the music therapist's bodies and minds are engaged in making new moments of relational experience.

I have come to believe as music therapists we are well-placed to deal with adoptees' non-verbal unconscious material because when we seek to attune to clients in embodied improvisational music-making, the medium of music, via its own special elements, can allow both body and mind to speak and to be heard. This basic rationale has underpinned the evolving psychoanalytic, attachment-based, trauma-informed, embodied, relational music therapy approach I have evolved. This overarching approach within client-led music therapy enables lived experience to emerge and be thought about and leads to sense-making in new ways which can enable the emergence of new relational possibilities. This is what happened for Joe.

Embodied affect-led music relating

Neuroscience has evidenced that embodied states created in past experiences might express emotional, relational affects in the here-and-now. Musical relationships, which occur in and through bodies playing together can express such affect wordlessly. Embodied memory, to be truly understood, needs to be felt and my work with ten-year-old Shayla certainly taught me to feel.

Shayla's memory

Shayla demonstrated embodied memory in a visceral way. She was referred because she experienced daily outbursts of extreme distress, becoming inconsolable. In contrast, in music therapy, Shayla could not make sounds at all and simply needed to sit silently and look at me. My supervisor suggested gazing together at each other might partially meet attachment needs such as the early gaze lost to Shayla. This could be the start of an attunement process.

Prior to adoption, Shayla had a history of abuse and neglect. Exploring my transference feelings arising as we silently gazed at one another, I realised I felt like an inadequate mother, unable to give or do anything useful in music therapy. This paralleled how her second mother felt too, who was despairing of ever really bonding with Shayla.

One day Shayla inadvertently knocked a beater off a xylophone. It made a single sound as it fell to the floor. Spontaneously I took up the remaining beater and played a single-note response. Shayla picked up her dropped beater . . . and played the next note . . . and I the next. We had finally begun a musical relationship. Shayla led our weekly music-making from this point on in this manner, always commencing with "accidentally" dropping a beater. She now also connected with early memories of her removal from her first family (which had felt like being "dropped") that could now be thought about safely.

Video recordings of sessions showed the "dance" of attachment and attunement developing between us. Though I never consciously or deliberately matched or mirrored my movements to hers, frequently a symmetry existed between us. The music that flowed out of embodied states was intimate and close, naturally matched and mirrored. Sletvold (2014) has described how within this flowing state, the ability to experience both similarities and differences between bodies constitutes the basis for the registration of significant affective experiences that emerge in a relationship. These registrations take place without the involvement of reflective thought or traditional forms of symbolic representation. We never spoke directly of Shayla's early lived experience, but memories were evident and could safely be enacted and considered.

Rhythms of relating: enabling intersubjective embodied music

The psychoanalyst Reich (1949) stressed the relevance of the creative arts in understanding the pre-linguistic nature of emotional experience and expression. The pre-verbal separation trauma known by all adoptees is one such pre-linguistic experience. Reich writes positively of music, stating that it can give expression to the inner movement of the living organism. He suggests that listening to music evokes the sensation of some earlier stirring because the beginnings of living functioning lie much deeper and beyond language. He acknowledges that although music is wordless, it yet has a capacity to enable deep feelings which can be shared in different bodies, which is identical to having contact beyond the limitations of language. I would add that as well as listening to music, the involvement of two human embodied people actually playing music together is wordless "self-embodied-in-relationship" and can be therefore potentially revealing of unconscious memory.

Joe's memories and meaning-making

I opened this chapter with a discussion of one memory of Joe's which emerged through his use of pop songs. While playing pop, Joe would engage in the typical postures of a young male pop star, yet I had an overwhelming sense of him as a vulnerable baby. As we worked with his songs, Joe engaged in sense-making, thinking that he might somehow be singing about himself. Eventually, we did have conversations about what was known of his early lived experiences. Joe already held these memories within his body and brought these to therapy unprocessed. Then, a combination of the musical elements and an attuned sensitivity to his material led to a profound shift of memory from unconscious to conscious awareness. Also, these songs, despite seeming adolescent, could offer Joe experiences of being held and rocked, that his baby self never experienced.

The next two narratives from my work highlight musically embodied communications of clients and how they were managed at the time. They illustrate why, when memory is being evoked, as the music therapist I must be alert to my own processes and exposure of any personally painful material. This is especially true as I share lived experience of adoption which can resonate usefully at points with clients but which needs to be processed and consciously held.

Katy's memories merge with mine

Katy was playing the piano and singing a song she made up about the physical abuse she had experienced in her first family which had resulted in scarring on her arm. I sat alongside her, supporting her melodic expressions with sustaining chords. Katy sang about being injured by her first mother, resulting in her scars. Then she sang that not only did she know that I could see her scars, but also sang, "You know because you have scars too." Katy had no knowledge of my own adoption narrative yet somehow had unconsciously tapped into it, linking our memories. I continued to hold the music while thinking of a response and gradually introduced a counter melody line with the words "you have scars too," as a way of recognising some similarity between us and our memories, but also stressing our difference so that the risk of any unhelpful merging was reduced.

George's memories shut me out

At the age of 16, George had secretly traced his first sister and, subsequently, his first mother via social media. First sister was delighted to be "found" by him and helped him to search for their first mother, who, once found, rejected both of them totally. George had not told me this happened but came to a session and drummed continuously, furiously and loudly, refusing to let himself be found at all in the music. I experienced his music as extremely painful and rejecting to receive and hold. In supervision, aspects of my own lived experiences and memories of rejection were identified honestly. Then I was able to share with George the sadness I felt at being shut out of his music, which had previously been relational. George sang, "Well, I'm shutting you out because she shut me out!" He then revealed his secret finding of and rejection by his first mother.

Then we involved his second mother in some shared music-making wherein she was able to help him manage painful feelings. Later, she encouraged him to try again to meet his first mum, but this time with support and stability.

Music therapy as embodied play where memories present

The music therapist Sami Alaane writes:

> Music is not an object; rather that I feel, hear and sing music *with my flesh. My body is the object that is felt, heard and sung*. The music reveals life in itself . . . we perceive and know the world subjectively through our bodies.
>
> *(Alaane, 2016, p. 15)*

This quote seems to describe embodied play in music therapy. Similarly, the words of the poet T.S. Eliot (1943): "You are the music, while the music lasts." Both quotes recognise that music exists only ever in a temporal, ephemeral form *while we are making it with our active bodies*.

In art therapy, clients create images which are tangible not just in the therapy room but also when taken by the therapist to supervision. Music does not exist outside of the original experience of playing it in the same way, even when it is recorded. Listening back to an experience makes the act of listening itself a memory, separated by time from the original experience. Embodied musical relationships can exist in time and space only. Music therapy then provides a *total embodied temporal experience* where memories can be revealed, addressed and survived. Feelings in the music therapist's body might then be identified as their own, or as projected material from the client. Joint music-making in music therapy requires my presence, which must be ever alive to an awareness of the *quality* of relationships *in the present time*. Music similarly exists in present time and this is important with regards to attunement. As Stern (2004, p. xiii) describes it:

> The present moment I am after is *the moment of subjective experience as it is occurring*, not as it is later re-shaped by words. What is shared in a moment of meeting is an emotional lived story. It is physically, emotionally and implicitly shared not just explicated.

The qualitative musical feel of implicitly shared intersubjective relationship is experienced in harmonic and rhythmical attention that involves the subjective felt senses of both client and therapist, encountered in what we so simply call "playing together." Adoptees might seek to silence me, or threaten my self-agency or deny that anything might be available for them in our musical relating. By controlling playing, choosing instruments, telling me how to play, dictating rhythm, etc., adoptees can either idealise or violate me as a therapist. But, when I survive such projections and am eventually able to play separately, as a self-in-relationship, a sense of musical conversation emerges. We gain a sense of an adoptee's earlier memories of relational experience. Then we can develop our own new reparative experience within music therapy, with the implicit aim of the adoptee being enabled to take this experience out into their wider world.

I need at times to play with intensity, but equally must be able to regulate my own playing, experimenting musically with closeness and distance within intersubjectivity. Wilkinson (2010) describes a "look/look away" interaction involved in sharing a visual gaze that people with attachment difficulties must feel in control of in psychotherapy. This is because the continued gaze of the therapist can be too much to bear at times, as within such gaze early memories may be evoked. Similarly, in music therapy, I need to balance sound-making or musical-gazing (looking) with silence (looking away). Then adoptees can lead the way in sense-making about new memories of warmth, similarity and empathy experienced within musical intersubjectivity.

Music therapy as embodying memory of the maternal

Jack's memories of mummy in music

Three-year-old Jack entered the music therapy room and stood opposite me, looking at me across the keyboard. He could reach all of the keyboard, which in his perspective was upside-down, and so we were immediately physically mirrored in our position. He began by soundlessly stroking the instrument's keys. It is impossible to play any musical instrument without bodily involvement; therefore, playing is always automatically an embodied experience. While mirroring Jack's embodied state, I also mirrored his gesture, similarly stroking the keys. Gradually, I increased my pressure, putting weight into my touch, then actually playing the keys, albeit very softly. Jack immediately looked up at me and whispered, "Mummy." Something in this shared, musically mirrored and embodied state had resonated something of an early maternal memory for him. He asked me then for a "Mummy song," which I was required to improvise.

I set up a repetitive chord sequence, this time using three chords of C/F/G major, in a slow 6/8 time. This pattern became an ostinato (this is a musical form which many adopted children have either requested from me or discovered for themselves) and over this, Jack began to sing repeatedly the word "mummy." I sang back this time, "Jack is here today in music with Joy." The repeating chord structure, held within a steady rhythm, could offer Jack a sense of regularity and certainty both musically and relationally. Many small but extremely significant interactions between a mother and her infant are repetitive (feeding, for example, has a regular repetitive rhythm).

Jack gazed intently at me throughout our play, which felt replicative again of the gaze between mother and infant. His body rocked rhythmically with my playing, and I found myself manifesting similar slow rocking in my own body, unconsciously, in reaction to his felt memory. We were resonating together as I/the music became a symbolic maternal object Jack could now use.

Very suddenly, Jack became tearful, now crying, "Mummy" quite loudly. I played and vocalised, adapting the music to his feeling tone. I then experienced a transferential need within myself to move physically closer towards Jack as a supportive presence. At this moment, I felt a strong countertransference of not being able to be "good enough." I doubted the simplicity of this music was adequate or that it could hold such intense memory, and so moved my body to get nearer to Jack. I then immediately wondered if my experience resonated with Jack's first mum's feelings. She had a learning disability and had not always been able to get it "right" for him. She had provided some initial attunement for Jack, but inconsistently, to the point that she was deemed unable to adequately care for him. Was I, simultaneously in transference, becoming like Jack's second mum and fearful that what I could provide would not be able to be received by him?

When I shared these feelings a few days later in supervision, my supervisor felt that Jack's sudden change of emotion and real distress came from a deeply felt early memory. My supervisor felt Jack did gain something emotionally from my closer physical repositioning and that the type of music I was playing was exactly that which was being called for. This music, albeit simple, was existent in the space between us and adequately holding Jack psychologically. I was able to continue to attune to Jack's vitality effects, inducing a reverie state.

As Jack cried the word "mummy" I sensed this memory was more about the loss of the attachment he had so briefly enjoyed, possibly, in the earliest moments of attunement with his first mum, but still held in his body memory. When Jack became upset, he would quickly become distressed and bereft. His eyes and nose would both run, with him making no attempt to dry them. He would stand, arms by his side, looking completely dejected. Perhaps this was why I felt so strongly the need to get nearer and offer physical comfort. However, these were also important feelings to allow space for. As I sang, "Jack is here in music today with Joy," I believed the music, as a temporal form, was evoking a painful past sensation while also safely holding us in Stern's here-and-now moment. Remembering the past was painful, and I did not want Jack to be flooded entirely by unconscious memory sensations. My words, therefore, orientated us both to the new experience he was simultaneously having here-and-now. There was a constant, fluid, ongoing conversation between conscious and unconscious aspects of Jack within the music and relationship. Time past and time present co-existed.

Much of this work, drawing on memory and holding it musically, has often felt to me as if a state like Bion's (1963) reverie is being created. Winnicott (1971) did not use the term reverie himself but defined a similar special state of receptivity to the infant, located within the mother in the earliest days of life that he calls primary maternal preoccupation. I have been enabled to hold Jack and others in varying states of reverie or with something akin to maternal preoccupation. As the adoptee client feels held, they can relish symbolic maternal presence if the therapist can manage to be with them in a non-invasive way, allowing their own personality to emerge.

We have thought then through this chapter about how adopted clients carry an internalised knowledge of early trauma which can manifest in music therapy as "the old present" – a term described by Wilkinson (2010). Almost all adoptees I have worked with have at some point acted out play involving ghosts, as experienced also by music therapist Robarts (2014). We know that difficult early experiences are embodied, and neuroscience informs us that strong emotions remain principally stored in the amygdala, unavailable to recall, yet governing ways of being and behaving. Such experiences have often entered the music therapy room in the form of "ghosts" as I describe now.

Charmaine's memories as ghost

Charmaine was seven when she began music therapy. In her first session, she formed an immediate connection with a large gong and played softly on it with a beater, creating a spooky atmosphere. She gently created layers and waves of sound in gradual crescendo, until the room was filled with vibrations. It felt mysterious yet safe, as if a warm musical mist was surrounding us. As she did this, I provided a consistent, enduring piano bass octave, rocking along in time with her gong. There was a thickness to the sound quality which felt representative of a feeling tone.

Suddenly Charmaine jumped backwards, exclaiming, "Did you see that?" and rushed to the opposite side of the gong to hide. I said I hadn't seen anything but was curious to know her experience. She shrugged and said, "Maybe it was a ghost?" This play repeated over many weeks, with this same build-up of a musically dense atmosphere, out of which things did seem to emerge, almost as shadows coming out of our musical mist. I supported this process on piano. Charmaine then began to sing of a 'ghost baby' that she could hear crying. Although the baby was never identified, Charmaine seemed very sad as she sang. This sadder feeling tone first needed acknowledgement and holding.

Then after some weeks of holding the sadness, I instinctively felt my own music changing, as I began playing in 6/8 time, that classic lullaby rhythm again. Charmaine's body began to rock in time, as though the piano music was holding her body memory of loss. As she rocked, I wondered about her internal baby and that baby's longing for the birth mother. Perhaps that "ghost baby" was also now musically held and could be comforted here and now? Charmaine's embodied rocking enabled her to soothe herself too and embrace the abandoned little baby she had been. She longed to feel securely attached to her adopted mother, but her "ghost baby" painfully reminded her that mothers could abandon. We never spoke about this, but the symbolism did its work. In later sessions, Charmaine's second mum wrapped her in a blanket, holding her like a baby, physically re-creating moments of early life that had been lost to them. Throughout their enactments, I sustained the piano lullaby. From this recapitulation of an early state, new, more secure relating could now emerge.

Conclusion . . . and a hopeful hypothesis

In my work in recent years, I have been exploring this hypothesis: that music therapy can provide a way for adoptee and therapist to become aware together of the client's previously unrepresented experience and embodied memory. Memory of experience can be revisited and taken from "then" to "now." Therapist and client play in the here-and-now and yet are simultaneously playing with earlier versions of the client's self (which has been both lost and found within the adoption process). The experience of being removed from the first mother happened when no one was there to witness and make meaning of such experience for the baby. Therefore, the adoptee carries an internal presentation that has been felt but not yet represented. This is why children who were unable to have *thoughts* about what was happening to them need to find *acts* to express their felt experiences. Affects can be transformed in both music and play. Then, what one of my PhD supervisors termed "the un-past" (Williams, 2021) can be turned into a historical past and meaning made of it.

I have come to understand this experience of the recall of the earliest of memories in terms of Freud's *après-coup*. This sense was first described by Freud as "Nachtraglichkeit." Later, it was translated by Lacan as "*après-coup*" and by Laplanche as "afterwardsness." I think that the *après-coup* feels similar to the notion of Plato's anamnesis stated earlier in this chapter. I have described, by use of the clinical vignettes in this chapter, how in my work there is often a sense of experience occurring 'here-and-now' in the music therapy room that brings back something, enabling us to make sense of early experience. I can pick up on affect in the music and understand symbolic play as often being rooted in early memory. As adoptees have new experiences of being held and cared for (both in music therapy and most significantly within their adoptive families), they can test me out to see if I can bear the repetition of their trauma. *Après-coup* is meaning that comes after an event. The "first experience" for an adoptee is their relinquishment by the first mother. The "second experiencing" is the *après-coup* which helps the first to be known. Adoptees can have this second experience with their second family but may only be able to reject care. I have hypothesised in my PhD that in music therapy a third "experiencing" occurs, which can give meaning to earlier experiences in both first and adoptive families. In this third experiencing, early memory of experiences can be enacted, symbolised, represented and then thought about and thereby gain meaning.

Adult adoptees who experienced the pre-verbal trauma of being removed from their birth mother as tiny babies often describe their enduring sensation of tremendous loss and separation. But adopted children lack the language to do this, especially those with additional special needs. Such pre-linguistic experience needs symbolic representation then because the traumatic experience came before language, and the creative arts therapies are well-placed to provide this. Music, not being reliant upon words, can connect with the adoptee's inner sensations, thus evoking pre-linguistic stirring and expression of feeling that is incapable of being put into words. Therefore, I argue that the experience of two human embodied people actually playing music together can potentially reveal to both a level of pre-verbal unconscious material. Old memory is safely held and new memory created. This is the hope of music therapy in adoption.

References

Alaane, S. (2016). *Music Therapy with Refugee Survivors of Torture*. Helsinki: Picasct Oy.

Bion, W. (1963). *Elements of Psychoanalysis*. London. Heinemann.

Eliot, T.S. (1943). *Four Quartets*. New York: Harcourt.

Freud, S. (1920/2003). *Beyond the Pleasure Principle: And Other Writings*. London: Penguin Classics.

Phillips, A. (1994). *On Flirtation*. Cambridge, MA: Harvard University Press.

Reich, W. (1949). Cited in Sletvold, J. (2014) *The Embodied Analyst: From Freud and Reich to Relationality*. Oxford: Routledge.

Robarts, J. (2014). Music Therapy with children with developmental trauma disorder. In C. Malchiodi and D. Crenshaw (eds.), *Creative Arts and Play Therapy for Attachment Problems*. New York: The Guildford Press.

Sletvold, J. (2014). *The Embodied Analyst: From Freud and Reich to Relationality*. Oxford: Routledge.

Stern, D. (1998). *The Interpersonal World of the Infant*. London: Karnac Books.

Stern, D. (2004). *The Present Moment in Psychotherapy and Everyday Life*. New York: Norton.

Sutton, J. (2002). *Music, Music Therapy and Trauma: International Perspectives*. London: Jessica Kingsley Publishers.

Trevarthern, C. (2009). In C. Trevarthern and S. Malloch, *Communicative Musicality: Exploring the Base of Human Companionship*. Oxford: Oxford University Press.

Verrier, N. (1993). *The Primal Wound*. Baltimore, MD: Gateway Press.

Williams, A. (2021). PhD supervision, 30th July. Zoom conversation.

Winnicott, D. (1971). *Playing and Reality*. London: Tavistock Publications.

Wilkinson, M. (2010). *Changing Minds in Therapy: Emotion, Attachment, Trauma and Neurobiology*. London and New York: Norton.

7

WORKING WITH MEMORY

The Making and Breaking of Personal Myths

Alanah Garrard

Abstract

This chapter examines how the phenomenological practice of dramatherapy and working with autobiographical memory allows one to address identity and a sense of self held in the stories and personal myths that have developed throughout our lives, particularly within our early developmental years. It is either through our memories of childhood or through the stories, memories and perceptions of others that are reflected to us, that we begin to form a sense of ourselves, who we are and the relationships that we form.

How does the perception of ourselves and our memories change as we travel through our lives and what can that teach us? What stories are we told by those around us that become part of these memories and form our idea of who we are? As dramatherapists, how do we work with the client's memories and how can this be done with the client's therapeutic objective at the forefront?

Using both theory and client material, I explore the role of memory and the experiences that form our personal myths, our perception of these as we develop throughout our lives and how dramatherapy can facilitate the making and breaking of our personal myths. It considers how dramatherapy can be envisioned as a phenomenological practice influenced by the philosophy of Merleau-Ponty in terms of embodiment, language and perception, how we are influenced through our pre-reflective consciousness (Sartre 2003) and how dramatherapy practice can aid in the existential issues of being-in-the-world and being-with-others (Heidegger, 1962).

Keywords: dramatherapy, phenomenology, memory, identity, body memory

DOI: 10.4324/9781032663944-7

Permission was sought and granted for all individual client work that is described in the following chapter.

A desire to understand oneself can potentially be the springboard that propels someone into seeking therapy. Some come to therapy in order to unravel the narratives of their lives and as a way of understanding their experiences, to consider choices they have made and the relationships that inform these in all parts of their lives and to try and make sense of these. In this chapter, I will be exploring how when we work with a client's autobiographical narrative and memories, we are working with their sense of self and identity, formed in the early years of their lives. I will consider what I mean by the term 'personal myth' and how memory and its applicability as a form of content in therapy informs our developing sense of self. I will reflect on Sartre's concept of the "original project" (Sartre, 2003) that begins in our early development as pre-reflective consciousness and will use examples drawn from my client work to consider how the phenomenological practice of dramatherapy can assist in the client's awareness of these personal myths in order to accept and embody them or reject and be released from them. One dramatherapy practitioner described the practice as one that "frequently privileges non-verbal, symbolic and metaphorical means of expression, thus foregrounding qualitative, and poetic aspects of human experience" (Pritchard, 2019, p. 18). The focus on the individual's embodied experience through creative expression offers space in which to explore the more concretised beliefs around early formed identity.

Philosophers have long ruminated over the power of memory. How do we know that a memory is a representation of the past rather than created from imagination and that the feeling associated with the memory is rooted in the past rather than a present representation associated with the memory (Blackburn, 2016)? Memory is a subject that has created and continues to create theories of construction, perception, realism and embodiment, to name a few.

> Memories are not really representations of something that happened but are schemas and engrams that form as a result of the mixing together of events and their social context, our psychological state, our mood and emotions, the environmental context, and our interactions with others.
>
> *(Caldwell, 2012, p. 258)*

Le Doux explains that each time we recall a memory, it becomes vulnerable to change and is in a labile state in which the altered version then gets reframed as the memory and carried forwards (Paulson *et al.*, 2013). Historically, psychoanalysis suggested that we can repress memories that stay intact until they may or may not return, and Schacter would agree that some memories can coexist with a reasonable degree of accuracy while there is also evidence that some memories become distorted through reconsolidation and the influence of our experience (Paulson *et al.*, 2013). I would suggest that as we look back at periods of our lives, our development and our experience can alter our understanding of a memory rather than the memory itself be changed. We look through a different lens, for example, when revisiting memories of our childhood, when we ourselves become parents, and when our understanding of what happened can change. At a discussion held at the New York Academy of Sciences on November 14, 2012, Winter stated that:

> it seems to me that memories are only perfect if one doesn't move on, if one doesn't live. And if you live, then you're changing . . . it is in this sense memory or self can be seen as an active dynamic thing.
>
> *(p. 45)*

In the title of this chapter, I have used the term personal myth, specifically the making and breaking of these as a focus within the therapeutic work, and for the purpose of this chapter, I will define what I mean by this terminology. One's personal myth is a subjective creation formed through psychobiological development that informs a sense of self and identity. It is formed from both conscious and unconscious material, (influenced by family systems and history, early development,) and throughout one's life that impact our choices and relational experiences. It can both bind us to who we believe ourselves to be and what we feel capable of, as well as provide a belief system that underpins how we choose to live:

> who we take ourselves to be dictates how we set up our lives individually and as a collective . . . early experience moulds behaviours, emotional patterns, unconscious beliefs, learning styles, relational dynamics, and the ability to handle stress and regulate ourselves.
>
> *(Mate & Mate, 2022, p. 124)*

But what happens when an event undermines a memory that in some way has formed into a truth, an understanding that underpinned a belief system, a way of being? The perception of a memory can become destabilised. This may occur through important life events such as moving away from home and meeting new people, a relationship ending, losing a loved one, becoming a parent or losing financial security. The list of possible changes that can be encountered, by choice or by chance, is extensive. As therapists, can we assist a client in addressing their sense of identity that has encountered some form of challenge, where long-held beliefs of their life story and relationships no longer hold true? What happens when our identity, formed through our memories, relationships and perceptions no longer feels congruent with the person we understand ourselves to be? Our belief system can feel challenged, we can fall into an existential crisis, no longer guided by the stories that grounded our identity, no longer fitting the narrative that we have told ourselves. This new perspective can leave one's memories feeling distorted, and misunderstood; but if we can work through this rocky terrain, it can lead to a clarity or path previously unseen. Dramatherapy is "a methodology [. . .] appropriate to lived embodied experience" (Pritchard, 2019, p. 19). It is a therapeutic approach that can assist through the art form of unravelling and reforming who we believe ourselves to be.

Client R lost her father to a sudden illness. She was one of four children and her parents were still married when he died. In the early days after this death, it came to light that he had been having a long-term affair with another woman. He had always taught the children that family and honesty were critical to living a good life. These two imperatives had been the cornerstone of their family ethos. This new information, discovered upon his death, threw everything that had underpinned her value system into disarray, and it took almost a year of working together before R could even begin to get in touch with her grief. For the first year, everything she felt she understood about her life and her family felt shattered. How much therefore of anything she believed in was real? She missed her father terribly but struggled to balance, on the one hand, the anger around the untruths and the false image portrayed, and on the other, her grief. We worked with story, the retelling of her stories, of her childhood and of who she and her father were in these. We worked with the imagery and sense of space around the home and country that she grew up in, the smells and sounds of the sea and the vista of the walks that she went on with her father to connect in an embodied way to her feelings of loss and anger. This use of imagery and movement gave her a form of expression that she could not find through words. As she revisited the significant memories and images of her childhood, she discovered that her father was, in many ways, still the father that she knew, and the shattered symbolic image of him had to be reformed in a new way:

> when we remember, we bring the past into the context of the present, and as that past surfaces it is exposed to the different experiential elements residing in the here and now. If these new elements are safe, calm, welcoming and relationally secure (i.e., a therapeutic relationship) a painful memory can be consciously worked with on a body level.
>
> *(Caldwell, 2012, p. 261)*

Part of recording a memory and what we store about our experiences are our perceptions and inferences at the time of the event that directly influence how we remember something (Paulson *et al.*, 2013). In the case above, client R was able to revise and realign her memories of her father once she had recovered from the shock and worked through her grief and anger. We reflected at the end of our work together how the significance of the seasons had been altered through her experience. Her father died at the beginning of spring and we started working together shortly after. As spring began the following year, it filled her with anxiety, sadness and anger at her continuing struggles. As we began to work towards our ending (as spring came around for a second time) it became apparent how different she felt emotionally, but also how she sensed a new beginning, a new formation of herself and of the relationship she had with her father which felt hopeful.

"Narrative is a human being's most important mode of autobiographical meaning-making. It is the language of our identity" (Brockmeier, 2015, p. ix). So how do our autobiographies develop? From early developmental milestones, through our school years, early romantic encounters, development of our relationship with work and those around us and our interactions with loved ones and acquaintances, all these parts create the story of our lives and as we develop through life, they help us form the sense of who we might be. Time and memory are interwoven. It is from this ongoing dynamic between time and memory that our autobiographies are born. Teske (2006) speaks of the neuropsychological functions that are involved in constructing the narratives through which we sculpt our identities. These functions include memory, emotional marking and temporal sequencing. He goes on to explain that we develop our capacity for autobiographical narrative via socialised emotional patterns, that, "our inner subjectivities, and even the boundaries of our individuality, are socially constructed and maintained" (p. 172). We need not only our own memories, but our relationships with others, both past, present and future to uphold the narrative that we have constructed of ourselves. Merleau-Ponty (1964) considers the psychosocial relationship regarding development in his paper, *The Child's Relation to Others*, in which he reflects on how a child has been moulded by his environment:

> there is no moment at which you could grasp, in a pure state, his way of perceiving, completely apart from the social conditioning that influences him. Inversely, you can never say that the way in which a child structures his social environment is unrelated to the hereditary or constitutional dispositions of his nervous system . . . It is never simply the outside which moulds him; it is he himself who takes a position in the face of external conditions.
>
> *(p. 108)*

As a child develops, there is an increasing awareness that they are in a relationship with others and the world. Langridge (2005) explains that as a child develops an awareness of self and others, so do they develop their understanding that they are "living in the facial expressions of the other and are living the others will in their conduct" (p. 92).

Sartre considers our development beginning in terms of pre-reflective consciousness, one in which our experiences have no sense of temporality or context, they are not yet owned by the act of reflection. These experiences, as we develop, are then made sense of, and we begin to fix the world and our relationship to it (Adams, 2019). We are born into a family, or at least with some form of care, and into relationships, and through these we develop a sense of who we think we are in this world and our narrative begins:

> we start very early to impose, choose, patterns of coherence on our experiences and it is these that constitute what Sartre calls, depending on the translation, our original or fundamental orientation to the world, our original choice.
> *(op. cit., p. 98)*

This original choice, informed by all the experiences around us, begins to form our identity. Many of these experiences will be implicitly held, they will be embodied and out of our direct consciousness, "what he feels before he can think is a *powerful determinant of what kind of things he thinks when thought becomes possible*" (Liedloff, quoted in Mate & Mate, 2022, p. 124). We develop our orientation to the world, informed by and often defined by our early years, our adolescence and our early adulthood that has been organised into who we think we are. This may feel difficult to challenge or question, at times perhaps editing out or forgetting events that may conflict with the original project in order to hold on to the story of ourselves.

We translate the residue of our experiences that persists across time into tales of who we are, and we use them to review our lives. This complex mixture of personal knowledge that we retain about the past is woven together to form the biographies of the self that provide narrative continuity – a set of memories that form the core of personal identity. New memories are inevitably influenced by old memories and pre-existing knowledge. "Storying is active, made and fluid, not passive, given and fixed" (Adams, 2019, p. 177).

Fundamentally, therapy can be seen as a form of storytelling, an exploration of narrative that has contributed to our sense of self. Schacter (1996) explains that what we experience as autobiographical memory is constructed from not only specific episodic memories but also general events and knowledge from historical events. So, this autobiography that holds us and informs us of who we are is made up of not just our own memories, but the framing and retelling of stories from friends, families and colleagues, as well as informed moments through history that place our lives in some kind of temporal order; the before or after specific events that puncture our own episodic memory. Often, we learn about ourselves through the perception of others, and who we think we are can be greatly impacted by the roles that are given to us. Much of the therapeutic work that we do can be centred on the exploration of these roles and myths that have developed, often without our consent or conscious understanding, but which contribute to our self-narrative. In the therapeutic space I have heard many versions of this: "I wasn't kind to my sister," "I was a demon child," "Oh, I was very difficult when I was younger," "I was never considered clever, creative but not clever," "I was sweet, I didn't get angry," "I was always spikey, tricky, hard to be around" and on these labels go, of who we are or who we have been told we are, that form the sense of ourselves.

> Psychologists have come to recognize that the complex mixtures of personal knowledge that we retain about the past are woven together to form life stories and personal myths. These are the biographies of the self that provide narrative continuity between past and future – a set of memories that form the core of personal identity.
>
> *(Schacter, 1996, p. 93)*

Adams (2019, p. 178) writes, "the task of therapy is to find out how the past choices led to the current actions and then to future intentions." I would go further and suggest that as therapists we can also assist in enabling our clients to reflect, through their experiences, on what parts of themselves remain authentic to who they feel they are in the present, and to explore and question the myths that have governed their sense of self to date. Clients may come into therapy with feelings of great ambivalence about what could be framed as their original orientation. Through some life events, they may have discovered that perhaps what they thought they wanted, they did not. Who they thought they were is not quite as they imagined.

Client N came to therapy in crisis. He was in his late twenties and was just in the process of moving in with his girlfriend of two years. In his description of them, they were happy and she was very kind and sweet, so why was he experiencing extreme panic attacks as final preparations were being made? During one of our first meetings, he spoke to me of his privileged upbringing, his private education and his influential family and friends. He also spoke of his discomfort around spending money on himself, and that he was not a particularly nice child, often mean to his sister. He showed great sadness at not being a better big brother, and of hurting this woman who was excited to be moving in with him. When we reached a moment that connected with emotions, rather than cognition, he would respond bodily, his eyes closed, almost as if his not being able to see me would protect him. There would be long periods of silence and stillness and pain that felt important to witness and stay with: "the dramatherapist is challenged to attend to the (often) wordless, unconceptualized and above all living phenomena of the psyche in the moment of their arising" (Pritchard, 2019, p. 20). As the work progressed, we looked back at his childhood, too complex and intertwined (as they often are) to unravel fully here, but at its core, N believed himself to be cruel and uncaring, and to say anything that would be considered unkind was unthinkable and would fulfil his belief that he was simply a bad person. As an adult, N would often find himself in intellectual arguments, moral and ethical disagreements with his friends as this was the only form of conflict that was bearable to him. If he was unhappy or upset with anyone, he would use his intellect as a form of expression. It was too difficult to articulate his uncomfortable feelings believing these reflected his nastiness. Friends would become frustrated with his need for argumentative positioning along with his lack of emotional availability. To be able to relate in an honest way was unthinkable. As we explored his story of who he thought he was, the rigidity of his identity and the relationships that formed this, he began to explore the possibility of relating in a new way. He still would often close his eyes, but when they opened, he would look directly at me, less ashamed to offer his feelings even if they were difficult. Sartre called a moment of understanding and pure reflection "double nothingness" (2003, p. 488), a moment where this new perception freed you from the past and in turn freed you from your fixed future. This revelation is both hopeful and terrifying in turn.

Perception plays a part in our day-to-day experiences and our memories influence those perceptions. How can our memories not also be impacted by the feelings of the present, and does this present emotional context change the memory or just offer a new perspective? Can this new lens through which we look at a memory reveal more about ourselves and our relationships? Seeing memories in a new light enables the possibility of creating new understandings, "giving new meaning to old experiences can constitute in and of itself a new experience, and this experience again invites us to further investigations and interpretations" (Brockmeier, 2015, p. 119f).

Perception is where we are in relation to an object, whether that be a table, a person or a memory. Throughout our lives, our perceptions of who we are and who others are to us will change, so we re-examine our memories and come to new understandings of ourselves as we reflect on the moments that seem important. When a client says I have already worked through my relationship with, for example, my mother or my father in previous therapy, does that mean their feelings, reflections or memories will never change? In *The Routledge Companion to Phenomenology*, Walter Hopp writes on perception, "While each experience provides reasons to believe in the reality of what it discloses, each also stands open to correction by future experiences" (Luft & Overgaard, 2012, p. 151).

A memory coming into consciousness is a subjective phenomenon, so how can we experience these and uncover their meanings in a way that can assist in developing our sense of self through the art form, for example, dramatherapy? No memory is fully complete. Each memory has more to it than what is revealed in any single experience, each perspective will offer a different view. Working through a memory with another can offer a perspective that has not previously been considered. When working through an art form, one can respond not necessarily to the words but to what Daniel Stern terms the vitality form with which a memory is remembered. "When the vitality forms of the experience can be evoked, a whole experience can tumble out" (Stern, 2010, p. 127). Stern described this vitality as a product of the mind's integration of many internal and external events, as subjective experience and as phenomenal reality. This vitality can allow for the feelings and the body to take over from the words. One can work with the experience of being with a client using a description of the phenomena either witnessed or felt, rather than using interpretation. Phenomenology allows us to change the aspect with which we see things and relearn how to look at our world. To reflect in a phenomenological stance is to bracket out our assumptions and experience the phenomena in the moment with immediate perception. According to Thomas Fuchs (2013), body memory is formed during our development. Through the repetition of experience, a habit structure is formed with our actions and interactions becoming implicit body knowledge. This knowledge contributes to our sense of ourselves and identity as we hold the stories of who we believe ourselves to be. The body holds experiences that

> . . . blanket the environment like an invisible network which relates us to things and to people . . . from childhood on, forms of bodily interaction are established and constantly reactualized. It comprises the self and the others, the conscious and the unconscious.
>
> *(Fuchs, 2013, p. 461)*

Working with the body, in movement and away from cognitive retelling, allows for the body's felt understanding of the experience to be known. As Merleau-Ponty (2002) defines it, the lived body is itself the subject of perceptual experience . . . not simply the mind's understanding of perception. The self is active not just internally but through our relation to others and the world. Through movement we experience our being-in-the-world and our being-with-others (Heidegger, 1962), through story we find the roles that speak to us and we can see our being in ways that we may not recognise, as well as patterns that we do recognise and repeat. The nature of our identity is so embedded in relationships and memories, often implicit and out of our awareness. Much of a person's experience and its immediate meaning is outside of language (Langridge, 2005).

This attention to movement over words brings to mind one of a series of movement sessions I regularly facilitated for an all-female group. I would often gauge the women's state and energy levels presented via a focus before deciding exactly what I was going to do in these sessions and this particular week, I felt, there was considerable resistance to the idea of movement. This may have been due to there being a few new clients who were settling in, which had caused some unrest within the group. The group was quite fluid with women finishing their time in the facility and leaving, as well as new women joining. A lot of the time the members of the group were all in different places in terms of their therapy, the idea being the more senior members were able to support the newer members. After checking in and noticing that many seemed unlikely to participate in a movement session, I went to the office and collected their box of phones and asked each member of the group to pick a song from their music library, something that they wanted to share with the group, and asked if they could say a little about why they chose it. We agreed to go around the group with each member saying a few words (not everyone spoke) as to why they picked the song while I cued them up on the system, and then we danced. We danced to each song, whether it was upbeat 80s, slow and melancholic, house music or drum and bass, to list a few. We worked with our bodies to experience the feelings and thoughts not yet caught in conscious thinking (Pritchard, 2019), offering a different form of attention, allowing for the possibility of insight in the difference of experience in that moment. After we danced, we sat and reflected on what it was like to move to their songs in this group, in this place, to the music that meant something to each of them. Some contributed and shared, and some did not, but a few recognised they were in very different places now, working on themselves and their lives. The music reminded them of people and earlier times, their bodies were taken back to a memory, but one that was being recollected and reformed. Although the music was full of memories, it felt different. Dancing to the songs with these women had given them a newly formed experience and a new memory to go along with the original ones. It also allowed them all to experience something of each other and learn a little bit of history in a way that went beyond words that I hope helped contribute to a sense of cohesion and inclusion. Everyone had participated on some level and as a whole group we had shared moments of play, laughter, sadness, loss and hope. Some reflected through language, but we all met through our bodies. "Therapeutic modalities that involve the moving of memory, or bodily re-enactment, have such powers to access the unresolved material that many therapy clients want to explore and resolve" (Caldwell, 2012, p. 258).

Existentially our autonomy and freedom are essential, but we form meaning and identity from our connectedness to other beings and to the world. We hold our beginnings in our bodies. Pre-language, our experiences and our relationships are felt, attachments made or falter and we are considered easy or difficult, funny or naughty, acceptable or unacceptable among other descriptions. These ways of being, decided through the experience of others, are learnt before we have the words to make sense of them (Adams, 2019). Our pre-existing knowledge powerfully influences how we encode and store new memories. By working with a memory that has aided the development of a deeply embedded sense of identity with an alternative perspective, through the body and working phenomenologically by bracketing the assumptions of how we think we understand it, can this break the personal myths with which we view ourselves and the story of our lives?

Put very simply, phenomenology is the study of things shown and experienced. Husserl developed phenomenology as a way of researching the nature of an experience. It acknowledges the difficulty of separating the objective from the subjective, "phenomenology can talk about a life as lived from within" (Adams, 2019, p. 14). It aims to reach an understanding through description rather than explanation, and by working in this way we challenge our assumptions, how we see ourselves in the world and the myths by which we live.

Merleau-Ponty's method of analysis into our perceptual consciousness and how we understand ourselves was "a phenomenology that emphasises perception as the lived embodied experience of a human subject that is inextricably bound up with this world" (Phillips, 2013, p. 141). For Merleau-Ponty (1964) the body is the seat of perception, the vehicle for being-in-the-world. Actions and interactions formed during our development become implicit body knowledge, and this body memory conveys the past in the present with the body holding and communicating beyond words.

The Sesame method of dramatherapy is a practice grounded in analytical psychology that utilises several creative art forms accessing and working with both consciousness and the unconscious through embodiment, movement, drama and myth. It is a client-led approach, allowing space in which new phenomena can emerge with the therapist framing, containing and reflecting on the experience. A relational approach that allows the therapist to attune with the client, connecting intersubjectively. Through the art form and through the body, be it movement, play or story, the client can explore through experience the stories and ways of being that make up their autobiography in order perhaps to address how these have impacted their identity and sense of self. The art form allows space in which the client may experience, without overwhelm, the possibility of other. The client may embody and experience something that has felt previously unreachable or disallowed through learnt systems. The body is a key instrument that can be used when working with memory therapeutically, "the role of the moving, sensing, feeling and emoting body can now be seen as fundamental to the developmental structuring of and subsequent neurogenetic changing of memory" (Caldwell, 2012 p. 255). How the body experiences the shift and feels understanding through affect within the therapeutic relationship can have a profound and reparative effect.

The example below I believe captures this approach to dramatherapy, and how working creatively and therapeutically with story allows for a phenomenological approach to be held and developed. In this instance, the story I picked when working one-to-one was *Snow White and the Seven Dwarfs*. It was the relationship with Snow White and the dwarfs that I wanted to explore with the use of character to act as a form of distancing to work on themes of relating, but something else occurred that was unexpected, and was a reminder about holding the phenomenological stance of epoche (the bracketing of assumption). What I, the therapist, was expecting to be received through the content of the story was not what the client chose to work with, and their expressing the request of working with the dwarfs, and my attention to this allowed for a development of the therapeutic relationship. After the first telling, and for a further two weeks, we worked on images of the dwarfs created by the client through drawing and an embodiment of these through movement. There were reflections about the dwarfs reminding the client of parts of themself. In the third week, the client asked if they could create their own dwarfs and name them, drawing their characteristics and reflecting that these were more specific developed parts of themselves. Again, the characterisation seemed to form a boundary in which they felt safe exploring their identity. This client had formed a concretised view of how they saw themself and the way they felt perceived by others. These developed characters allowed them to, I believe, move their self-image from a rigid view to one that was more fluid and changeable as they played with the images. As the weeks progressed, we discussed the parts that made up the whole and the bits that they did and did not like about who they were and how they saw themself. Through working with a collection of projected images of their creation they were able to clarify which felt like real parts of themself and which felt like parts that were given to them. Had we not gone through the art form of story and image, I do not think that we would have reached such an open place of discussion around their identity and how they saw themself. It felt brave and open and allowed them to integrate not just the good but also the difficult parts of themself.

I hope, through the discussion above, I have outlined how memories both specific and non-declarative can contribute to an overall sense of self and identity, creating what I have termed for the purpose of this chapter one's personal myth, made up of both conscious and unconscious elements impacting all aspects of one's life. Through our psychological development these memories at times have "no words and no time stamp" (Caldwell, 2012, p. 257). They are both made up of past actions and remain in the present, with early experiences laying down "unconscious maps" (op. cit.). These maps are held as body memories and shape how we respond not only in the past but also in the present. According to Fuchs, phenomenologically the unconscious of the lived body is not intrapsychic but rather it surrounds conscious life. It is not in the vertical dimension of the psyche but in the horizontal dimension of lived space (Fuchs, 2013). Working therapeutically with the body and through creative art forms can allow us to attend to our clients' embodied states.

Relationships are fundamental to memory making, not just from our own perspective and experiences but those important early relationships that impact the beginnings of who we are and how we begin to define our identities. As a therapist in practice, the relationship I have with my clients and how I work, I hope, allows for a safe exploration of self, and the stories and narrative that make up their identity. Working through the art form and through a phenomenological approach that requires assumptions and interpretations to be placed to the side, it is my hope that what emerges through the client's exploration and understanding is who they choose to be, unencumbered by the myths that may have previously burdened them.

References

Adams, M. (2019). *An Existential Approach to Human Development*. London: Palgrave.

Blackburn, S. (2016). *The Oxford Dictionary of Philosophy* (3rd edn.). Oxford: Oxford University Press.

Boyle, A. (2020). The impure phenomenology of episodic memory. *Mind and Language*, 35, 641–660.

Brockmeier, J. (2015). *Beyond the Archive*. Oxford: Oxford University Press.

Caldwell, C. (2012). Sensation, movement and emotion: explicit procedures for implicit memories. In S. Koch, T. Fuchs, M. Summa, & C. Muller (eds.), *Body Memory, Metaphor and Movement*. Amsterdam and Philadelphia: John Benjamins Publishing Company.

Fuchs, T. (2013). Body memory and the unconscious. In R. Gipps & M. Lacewing (eds.), *The Oxford Handbook of Philosophy and Psychoanalysis*. Oxford: Oxford University Press.

Heidegger, M. (1962). *Being and Time*. Trans. J. Macquarrie & E. Robinson. Oxford: Blackwell Publishing.

Jones, P. (1996) *Drama as Therapy*. London: Routledge.

Langridge, D. (2005). 'The Childs Relations with Others' Merleau-Ponty, Embodiment and Psychotherapy. *Journal of the Society of Existential Analysis*, 16(1), 87–99.

Luft, S. & Overgaard, S. (eds). (2012). *The Routledge Companion to Phenomenology*. Oxon: Routledge.

Macey, D. (2000). *Dictionary of Critical Theory*. London: Penguin.

Mate, G. & Mate, D. (2022). *The Myth of Normal*. London. Vermilion.

Merleau-Ponty, M. (1964). *The Primacy of Perception*. Evanston, IL: Northwestern University Press.

Merleau-Ponty, M. (2002). *The Phenomenology of Perception*. Trans. C. Smith. Oxon and New York: Routledge.

Paulson, S., Aciman, A., LeDoux, J., Schacter, D., & Winter, A. (2013). The mystery of memory: in search of the past. *The Emerging Science of Consciousness: Mind, Brain, and the Human Experience*, 1303(1), 36–55.

Phillips, J. (2013). Merleau-Ponty and psychoanalysis. In R. Gipps & M. Lacewing (eds.), *The Oxford Handbook of Philosophy and Psychoanalysis*. Oxford: Oxford University Press.

Pritchard, W. (2019). Listening at the edge: attending to living process in Sesame dramatherapy. *Dramatherapy*, 40, 17–27.

Sartre, J.-P. (2003). *Being and Nothingness: An Essay in Phenomenological Ontology*. Trans. H.E. Barnes. London: Routledge.

Schacter, D. (1996). *Searching for Memory*. New York: Basic Books.

Stern, D. (2010). *Forms of Vitality*. Oxford: Oxford University Press.

Teske, J. (2006). Neuromythology: Brains and stories. *Zygon*, 4(1), 169–196.

8

MEMORY DRAWING FOR CHILDREN WHO HAVE EXPERIENCED STRESS AND/OR TRAUMA AND HAVE SPECIFIC LEARNING DIFFICULTIES

Unnur Guðrún Óttarsdóttir

Abstract

A study on memory drawing, regarding how emotions stemming from stress and/or trauma can be processed while simultaneously memorising coursework through such drawing is reviewed in this chapter. The aim of the research was to develop, study and test a therapeutic method that would facilitate emotional well-being and coursework learning for children who have experienced stress and/or trauma and have specific learning difficulties, such as difficulties with literacy, memorisation and mathematics. Five children who had experienced stress and/or trauma and had specific learning difficulties were selected for case studies. Grounded theory research methodology was applied in order to build an initial theory of the art educational therapy (AET) method that was developed. Memory drawing is a component of AET. Vignettes derived from the case study conducted with one of the children who participated illustrate how feelings of vulnerability stemming from memories of stress and/or trauma can be processed through memory drawing while simultaneously memorising coursework material. Indications were found that the unique integration of therapeutic work and coursework learning through memory drawing in AET has the potential to aid both emotional processing and containment, as well as in memorisation. The findings of the present study provide information for art therapists in schools who wish to incorporate memory drawing into their practice.

Keywords: trauma, children, memory, art therapy, art educational therapy (AET), coursework learning, emotions, memory drawing

DOI: 10.4324/9781032663944-8

Abstract in Icelandic

Í kaflanum er gerð grein fyrir minnisteikningu og eiginleikum hennar. Minnisteikning var rannsökuð í tengslum við úrvinnslu tilfinninga, sem stafa af álagi og/eða áföllum, um leið og námsefni er lagt á minnið með slíkri teikningu. Markmið rannsóknarinnar var að þróa, rannsaka og prófa meðferðaraðferð sem eykur tilfinningalega velferð og auðveldar nám barna sem hafa upplifað álag og/eða hafa orðið fyrir áföllum og eiga við sértæka námsörðugleika að etja, svo sem í lestri, stafsetningu, málfræði eða stærðfræði, sem og við að leggja námsefni á minnið. Til þátttöku í tilviksrannsókninni voru valin fimm börn, sem höfðu upplifað álag og/eða orðið fyrir áföllum og áttu við sértæka námsörðugleika að stríða. Rannsóknaraðferð grundaðrar kenningar var beitt til að móta frumkenningu um námslistmeðferðina sem þróuð var, en minnisteikning er liður í námslistmeðferð. Myndir teiknaðar af einu barnanna sem tóku þátt í tilviksrannsókninni sýna hvernig mögulegt er að vinna úr viðkvæmum tilfinningum tengdum minningum um álag og/eða áföll með minnisteikningu og leggja námsefni um leið á minnið. Vísbendingar fundust um að einstök samþætting meðferðar og náms með minnisteikningu í námslistmeðferð geti stuðlað að úrvinnslu tilfinninga og utanumhaldi þeirra og einnig að því að leggja námsefni á minnið. Niðurstöður rannsóknarinnar gagnast listmeðferðarfræðingum í skólum sem vilja innleiða minnisteikningu í starf sitt.

Introduction

Art therapy and memories of trauma

Psychological trauma can leave individuals feeling helpless as a consequence of overwhelming traumatic experiences. The internal caring system which provides a sense of control, connection and meaning is overwhelmed by the trauma (Herman, 2015). Traumatic stress results in the breakdown of children's capacity to regulate internal states (van der Kolk, 2007). The traumatised child needs to feel safe in therapy in order to process the traumatic experiences in therapy so that re-traumatisation does not take place (Karp and Butler, 1996; van der Kolk, 2007).

Although there is a shortage of evidence-based research on art therapy for traumatised clients (Schnitzer, Holttum and Huet, 2021), it is claimed to be an effective therapeutic method for traumatised children and adolescents, mostly based on case studies and practice (O'Brien, 2004; Eaton, Doherty and Widrick, 2007; Orr, 2007; Malchiodi, 2012, 2021; Ugurlu, Akca and Acarturk, 2016; Rowe *et al.*, 2017). Appleton (2001) proposed that hope can be found through art, and Kozlowska and Hanney (2001) stated that the art-making process facilitates a shift from feelings of helplessness to hope. According to Malchiodi (1998), the non-verbal quality of artwork has the potential to facilitate working through emotional trauma and associated emotions for which there are no words. Containment is facilitated through art-making in art therapy, where the artwork's boundaries (e.g., the borders of the paper) provide a concrete vessel that can contain fragmented traumatic experiences (Avrahami, 2006). Because the pain of trauma can be so overwhelming that words cannot explain it, it is easier for many children to use visual communication before talking about the trauma (Rubin, 1999). It is also claimed in the art therapy literature that traumatic experiences can be recollected through art-making (Meyer, 1999; Appleton, 2001; Eaton, Doherty and Widrick, 2007; Hass-Cohen and Clyde Findlay, 2019).

Trauma creates sensory memories, which art-making can reach better than verbal language (Talwar, 2007; Malchiodi, 2012). Memory reconsolidation (MR) factor is when the trauma memories are worked with in art therapy and thereby modified through the creative work in order to make them less distressing. Although there is limited research on this subject, Hass-Cohen, Bokoch and Julia's (2022) study found creativity to be an MR factor.

However, within the art therapy literature, there is a shortage of discussion about the possible limitations of art-making when working with traumatised populations. Laub and Podell (1995) discussed the importance of art-making in representing trauma, but at the same time, they proposed that art-making could reach too far and thereby cause unbearable emptiness to emerge. I suggest that integrating coursework learning, which refers to the children's schoolwork including mathematics, literacy, foreign languages and geography, into the art therapeutic work can provide an important contribution to art therapy for traumatised children. By integrating intellectual coursework learning into art therapy, including memorising, the traumatised child is offered time and means to gather cognitive strengths in order to further the ability to come to terms with, process and regulate vulnerable feelings relating to stress and/or trauma (Ottarsdottir, 2018b).

Other approaches also add to the cognitive and emotional integrative quality of art therapy, such as the art therapy trauma protocol (ATTP), where the client accesses traumatic memories through art-making while walking back and forth between the painting and the paint jars with the aim of activating dual processing of the left and right hemispheres of the brain. This method is based on bilateral drawing and Eye Movement Desensitisation and Reprocessing (EMDR), which are integrative approaches that engage both hemispheres of the brain when working with trauma memories (Talwar, 2007).

Edwards (2008) introduced the technique of "drawing on the right side of the brain," which includes certain drawing exercises designed to activate the right side of the brain, often by excluding verbal labels of the drawn object and concentrating on the form and the visual drawn line. One of the exercises that Edwards presented is to turn the drawn object upside down in order to exclude the verbal left-brain knowledge and instead focus on the lines and forms. This is in a way similar to the approaches of AET, where the visual and emotional functions are activated by the process of drawing in relation to the verbal and intellectual content of the coursework. One of the AET ways to more closely integrate the verbal/cognitive and the visual/emotional aspects is to write a word and then turn the word upside down, which is followed by tracing the lines of letters upside down.

The AET approach, developed through the present research, embeds the principles of trauma-informed practice and principles (Malchiodi, 2021). This includes understanding the way in which stress and/or trauma impact a child's well-being and coursework learning. Providing emotional containment and safety within the therapeutic relationship is an important factor in AET. The foundation of art therapy theories, i.e., that symbolic emotional material can be expressed through drawing (e.g. Edwards, 2004), is part of the theoretical framework for AET.

The focus of the present research was on the effect of stress and/or trauma on the inner life of the child and their coursework learning, with less attention paid to defining the situation as either stressful or traumatic. Instead of observing whether the child had or had not experienced trauma, attention was paid to whether there were emotions relating to difficult events in the child's life that had not been processed, integrated and worked through, which could have affected the child's emotional well-being and coursework learning.

Art therapy in education

Art therapy has been conducted within education since the early days of the profession (Cohen, 1975; Kramer, 1977). Various art therapists have reported on their work and research regarding art therapy in schools (e.g. Ratnik and Rüütel, 2019), and various systematic reviews have been conducted on the literature about art therapy in schools (e.g. Abramovski *et al.*, 2019; Frydman, Hyman and Caputo, 2022). Moula *et al.* (2020) completed a review of seven studies about art therapies in schools and found that the therapy had, according to the children, a positive impact on some emotional, behavioural and learning factors. McDonald and Drey (2017), who conducted a review of four research papers on the effectiveness of primary-school-based art therapy, found some positive effects of art therapy and no negative effects.

Harpazi *et al.* (2020) found, through in-depth semi-structured interviews with 12 adolescents who received art therapy in school, that the therapy helped them in various ways in relation to emotional factors. McDonald and Holttum (2020) focused partly on the link between art therapy and coursework learning, where they found no difference in terms of reading, writing and mathematics grades between the children who received art therapy and those who were in a comparison group. However, they reported that both children and teachers found that art therapy helped with coursework learning. A study conducted by Moula *et al.* (2023) revealed that school-based art therapy impacted the children's exploration of safe space, stress relief, emotional expression and empowerment in a positive way. However, the improvement did not reach statistical significance, possibly due to the small sample size.

Additional research studies which have not mainly focused on the effectiveness of art therapy in schools have also provided insights into the subject. For example, Deboys, Holttum and Wright (2016) conducted a grounded theory study in schools which indicated the importance of art therapy interventions in supporting children's emotional and social health. In a process-outcome study, Regev (2022) found that the process of school-based art therapy for children is more complex than is commonly believed for art therapy. Also, Regev, Green-Orlovich and Snir (2015) conducted a study which examined issues regarding integrating art therapy into schools. Their findings indicated that a greater knowledge of art therapy within the educational system would facilitate the practice of art therapy within the schools.

The findings of Adoni-Kroyanker *et al.* (2019), which included perspectives of 16 art therapists, showed that there is a gap between the reality of the educational system and the art therapists' practices and field training. They suggested that the training of school art therapists should be broadened in terms of modalities and models applicable to the educational setting.

Teachers and art therapists have cooperated in various ways. For example, art therapist Reddick (2008) worked alongside teachers within a classroom setting, and Ayalon (2021) introduced the Arts Therapist-Teacher model for arts therapists and teacher cooperation. In the Open Studio model, the teacher and the art therapist run the studio together (Regev, 2023). In addition, the integration of art education and art therapy took place within a programme conducted by the art therapist and art educator Albert (2010), where art therapy was combined with art teaching within the art educational classroom. Similarly, Dickson (2015), who is also an art therapist and art educator, integrated the theories and methods of art therapy into art teaching by, for example, introducing artwork made in art therapy sessions to the students.

Art Educational Therapy (AET)

The aim of the present research was to develop, study and test a therapeutic method which would facilitate coursework learning and emotional well-being. Memory drawing is part of the AET method developed through this study. To demonstrate a part of AET that relates to memory drawing, vignettes from one of the case studies conducted are presented in this chapter.

Theories of art therapy and educational psychotherapy created the theoretical framework of AET, along with the findings of the present research. Coursework learning is integrated into educational psychotherapy while the way in which emotional difficulties, including memories of trauma, can affect coursework learning is explored in-depth, together with how the therapy can facilitate such learning (e.g., Dover, 2003; Best, 2014).

In some of the AET sessions, the children spontaneously make artwork in an art therapeutic way, where the creative activity has free association and expressive qualities while it is not directed in any way by the therapist. The children spontaneously take the initiative, often without much conscious thinking, in terms of choosing to make art, what materials they use, what form the art takes, and what subject they work with. Other sessions include direct teaching, in which the therapist provides guidance and explanations in terms of specific coursework subjects. There are sessions where the method of integrating coursework into art therapy through art-making is applied, as the children make art in relation to their coursework learning in various ways. In numerous sessions, there is an overlap of approaches and a dynamic interplay between them. The children are encouraged to indicate what they would like to do in relation to coursework learning and art-making and they make their own choices in the sessions: to learn coursework, make art or combine the two in a variety of ways.

Containment, therapy, thinking and coursework learning

In the present study, one way to investigate the relationship between emotions stemming from stress and/or trauma and coursework learning was to observe the function of containment. Bion (1962b) has been cited both by art therapists (Case, 1990; Dalley, 2000) and by educational psychotherapists (Dover, 2002; Greenwood, 2002) in relation to containment. According to Bion (1962a), "containment" is defined as the process by which the child projects intolerable feelings onto the mother who, if she is capable, contains the emotions by receiving, accepting and understanding them, while she empathises, mirrors and returns the emotions in a tolerable form which subsequently facilitates the development of thoughts and a capacity to think. The therapist's task is similar to that of the mother: to contain the child's overwhelming unbearable feelings, thereby facilitating the ability to tolerate frustration and to think.

Case (2003) and Dalley (2000) claimed that art-making within the therapeutic relationship contributes to the containment of the child's emotions. Referring to Bion's (1962b) discussion of containment, Case (1990) explained that through containment the child develops a capacity to think, which can be a prerequisite for further learning.

Memory drawing

The term memory drawing has dual meanings in AET, which are linked to both drawing and memory. First, it refers to working with memories of life events by drawing in various ways. Second, it means applying drawing to memorise facts that can relate to coursework learning material. These two functions are related in terms of memorising and drawing, while the recollected content is different. The former definition, which relates to memories of life events, is to a greater extent related to art therapy, whereas the latter definition, which refers to working with memorising facts, refers more to education. In AET, those two ways of memorisation are often applied simultaneously within one and the same drawing.

Indications were found within case studies that drawing facilitated the memory of coursework. To investigate this further with a larger group of participants, 134 children participated in a quantitative study on the impact of drawing on memory. This quantitative study was linked to the qualitative case studies involving five children, in terms of the shared subject matter of memory drawing. However, the quantitative study was separate from the qualitative case study research design. Hence, the five children who took part in the case study did not participate in the quantitative part of the study (Ottarsdottir, 2018b).

In the quantitative study, a comparison was made between memorising written words and word content that was drawn. Recall took place immediately after memorisation, three weeks and nine weeks later. Drawing generally facilitates longer-term memory to a much greater extent than writing down words (Ottarsdottir, 2018b). Wammes, Meade and Fernandes (2016) also published their findings from a study that compared memory of written and drawn words over a shorter time period, where they too found that drawing the meaning of the words or their content was generally a more effective way to memorise words than writing them. Additional research has since confirmed that drawing is generally more effective for memorisation than writing (Wammes, Meade and Fernandes, 2017, 2018; Fernandes, Wammes and Meade, 2018; Meade, Wammes and Fernandes, 2018, 2019; Wammes, Jonker and Fernandes, 2019; Meade, Ahmad and Fernandes, 2020; Roberts and Wammes, 2021; Jalava, Wammes and Cheng, 2023).

Psychologists who have investigated memory and drawing have claimed that the reason for the effectiveness of drawing for memory is the integration of visual, motor and semantic information (Wammes, Meade and Fernandes, 2016) and that it creates contextual information that facilitates later recall (Wammes, Meade and Fernandes, 2018). In addition, from an art therapy viewpoint, the personal and emotional material implicit in the drawing is partly what makes it more memorable than written words which are generally more detached from the personal and emotional meaning (Ottarsdottir, 2018b).

Methods

Study design and data analysis

Case study research methodology was applied in order to study in-depth the complex individualised therapeutic and educational processes of the children who took part in the case studies in relation to the research questions posed (Yin, 2014). Because the data collected according to the case study research method was found to have many strands, grounded theory research methodology was applied to systematically analyse the data in order to build an initial theory of the therapeutic method developed (Strauss and Corbin, 1998). Drawn diagrams were applied to the grounded theory analytic process in order to deepen understanding and create concepts, as well as to investigate connections between phenomena, categories and concepts (Óttarsdóttir, 2013; Ottarsdottir, 2018a).

The symbolic meaning embedded in the artwork was analysed therapeutically, e.g., what the child may have been expressing symbolically when drawing the images. The therapeutic analysis was carried out according to psychodynamic art therapy frameworks, such as that images made in the therapy may have meaning that is helpful in understanding the client's state of mind (e.g. Edwards, 2004) and, according to Schaverien (1999), the drawing does not necessarily tell us something about the individual, but it indicates a possible analysis in relation to various aspects of the person.

Procedures and ethics

Material from unpublished parts of the case study of John (pseudonym) presented in this chapter demonstrates the way in which coursework learning, which includes memory drawing, can be integrated into art therapy when working with children who have experienced stress and/or trauma. Parts of the case studies have been reviewed in previous publications (Ottarsdottir, 2010a, 2010b, 2018a, 2018b, 2019).

John, who is now an adult, provided informed written consent for the anonymised use of his potentially identifiable images and other data for publication. This study was approved by The Icelandic Data Protection Authority.

Measurements and/or materials

The study was conducted in a small room in a secondary school in Iceland. Basic art materials were available for the children to use, including crayons, paint, clay, pencils and paper. Books related to the children's coursework learning were also available, such as dictionaries and textbooks on mathematics, spelling and grammar. In addition, the children brought their own coursework learning books and assignments to work within the therapy.

The five children who participated in the case studies received a total of 123 individual therapy sessions. John, who took part in the case study presented in this chapter, received a total of 32 sessions and he attended individual sessions twice a week over a period of one school year. The other children who took part in the other case studies received 18, 16, 16 and 41 sessions.

Participants

The five children who were selected for the case study had experienced stress and/or trauma. In addition, they had specific learning difficulties in terms of their school coursework, including mathematics, spelling, grammar, foreign languages and memorisation. The selection process included:

a. examination of school grades of children aged between 10 and 14;
b. interviews with school personnel about possible difficulties that the children who were selected because of low school grades may have experienced; and
c. examination of school reports in order to select children who had experienced stress and/or trauma.

In addition, the selection criteria included the children having:

d. adequate ego development;
e. sufficient family support; and
f. no evidence of developmental disabilities, brain damage, or drug or alcohol abuse (Ottarsdottir, 2010b, 2018b).

Vignettes from John, who was in therapy when he was 12 years old, were chosen for presentation in this chapter because they have a clear link to its focus, which is trauma work, memory drawing and memorising coursework.

Case study: John

Background information

At the age of 18 months, John's parents divorced. He and his mother then moved in with his grandparents who both later developed cancer. The mother took care of her ill parents and thus she may have had limited time and energy to take care of John. John's grandparents passed away around the time when he began going to school. The boy had been close to his grandparents. At the time of therapy, John seemed to miss his father.

When John was learning to speak, his parents divorced, which was followed by limited contact with his father. He was then affected by his grandparents' illnesses. Around the time when he was beginning to learn to read at school, his beloved grandparents passed away. When John began therapy, he had difficulties in terms of coursework learning, especially in terms of reading and spelling, and he was diagnosed with dyslexia.

Case study vignettes

Session VI

In this session, John wished to learn spelling. It can be difficult to decide whether to write i/í/ei or y/ý/ey in Icelandic because the letters sound the same. One way to know whether a word is spelt with i/í/ei or y/ý/ey is to find related words or the stem of the word. If there is "o," "u," or "ju" in the related word, the doubtful word contains "y," not "i." If the related word has "jó," "ú" or "jú" the doubtful word contains "ý" not "í." If the related word has "au" in it, the doubtful word is written with "ey." To facilitate memorisation of this spelling rule and possibly process some of his underlying emotional material, I suggested that John write "o, u, ju>y, jó, ú, jú>ý" and "au>ey" in big letters on an A4-sized piece of paper and then make images out of the letters (see Figure 8.1).

As John was drawing, he explained that the image on the top was a mother potato in the ground with baby potatoes growing out of her. The "u" below had been turned into a face. Underneath, liquid was poured into a glass. Below that were two men who had been fighting, then came a bath being filled with water and below that was an old weapon that had been used in war a long time ago. A Chinese person who owned the balls in the glass was at the bottom of the picture, along with a smiling man with a glass into which old wine was being poured.

Some of these images relate to nurturing. The first image is that of a mother potato nurturing baby potatoes. The two images of pouring a drink and running warm water into a bath may also relate to nurturing. The word "old" appears twice: an old weapon and old wine. There are also two people turning their backs on each other, with an old weapon nearby.

This was the only occasion when the themes of mothering (the mother potato), containment (letters used as containers), and nurturing (baby potatoes, the drink and warm water in a bath) were raised in the therapy. Possibly the nurturing presented in the drawing was related to the nurturing – including the containment – that he had or had not received. The nurturing provided by the mother potato (which may have symbolised his mother) at the beginning may somehow have turned into a weapon and fighting, which possibly symbolised disagreement and separation between his parents.

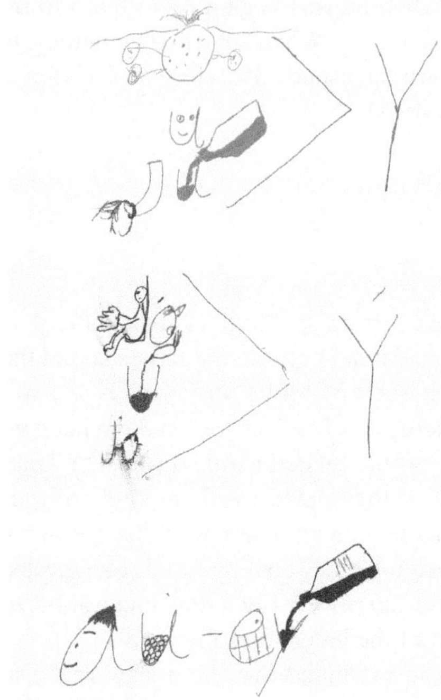

FIGURE 8.1 Memory drawing.

The mother had a difficult time when John was young because of her divorce and her parents' illness, and thus she may have been unable at times to provide the nurturing and containment he needed. This possible shortage of containment may, in turn, have resulted in some lack of thinking space, which possibly later contributed to John's specific learning difficulties, including memorising the way in which words were spelt in relation to the associated spelling rules.

John may have been working with feelings about the split between his parents as an "old" issue (old wine, people turning their backs on each other, and an old weapon). The last image shows two seemingly happy people and old wine being poured into a glass. John may have hoped that the therapy would make it possible for him to work through his "old" issues. He may also have hoped that his parents would get back together.

John used four letters as containers. On three occasions it was a "u," the first letter of the therapist's name. Perhaps he was considering the extent to which the therapist was able to contain his feelings. Maybe John realised on one level that language (the letters) could contain his emotions (symbolised by the liquid flow) and, like the therapist, art-making and coursework learning within the therapy could also contain his emotions.

After we discussed the content of the image, John recalled when to use "y," "ý" and "ey" by filling in letters that lead to "y," "ý" or "ey" (see Figure 8.2). He then practised further by putting "y" into words and writing the related words (see Figure 8.3).

Further on in the therapy, John wanted to practise the "y" spelling rule exercises again (see Figure 8.2). At first, he did not remember which letters lead to

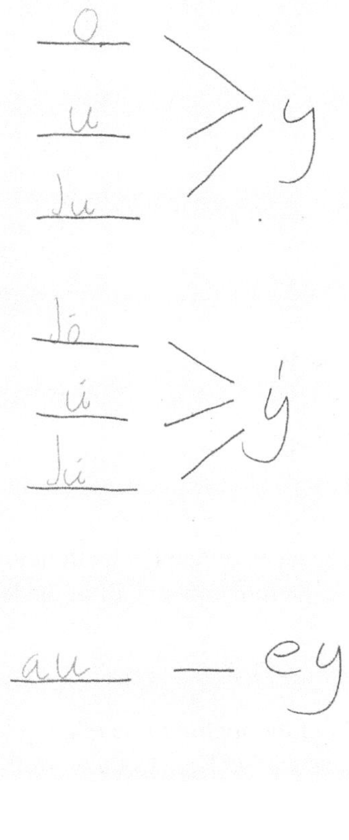

FIGURE 8.2

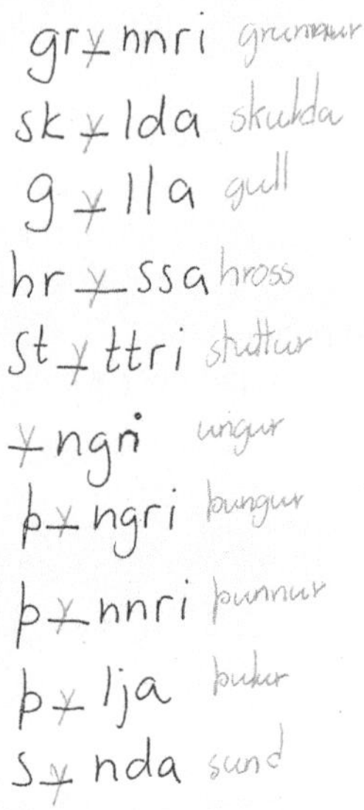

FIGURE 8.3

y/ý/ey, but when I suggested that he try to remember by thinking about the drawn images he had made in Figure 8.1, he remembered all of the letters correctly.

Session VIII

When John was learning more about the spelling rule relating to whether to spell words with i/í/ei or y/ý/ey, I suggested that he select a word from the dictionary with "y," which is related to the spelling rule and then draw its meaning. From all the words presented in the dictionary, he chose the word *yfirbugaðir* Icel. ("overwhelmed" in English). First, he wrote the word at the top of the page along with the related word, which was *of* Icel. ("too" in English) or *ofar* Icel. ("above" in English). He explained that the drawing in the middle of the circle was a machine surrounded by soldiers who had overwhelmed it, for example during the Second World War when soldiers overwhelmed Hitler's machines (see Figure 8.4). Perhaps John was expressing the emotional memory of being overwhelmed by the stress and/or trauma he had experienced in relation to his parents' divorce, the tiredness of his mother and the illness and loss of his grandparents, in addition to missing his father who lived abroad at the time of therapy and dealing with his specific learning difficulties.

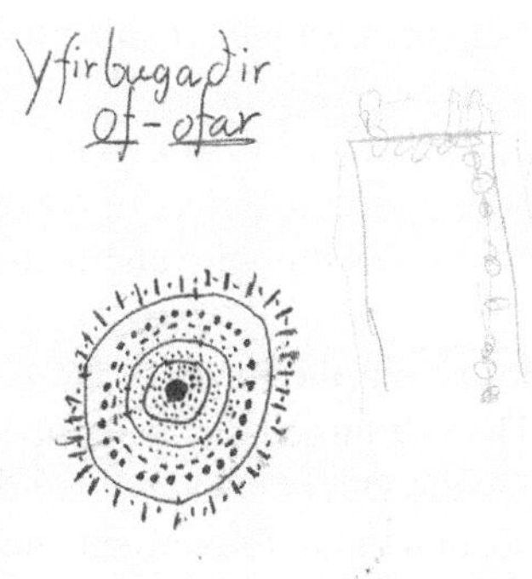

FIGURE 8.4 Memory drawing.

Session XIII

In this session, John was introduced to the method of writing upside down. I demonstrated the method to him using the following steps:

1. I folded an A4 piece of paper in half.
2. As I explained that I was drawing letterforms, I drew large letters on one half of the paper, making the word *LESTUR* Icel. ("READING" in English).
3. I then turned the piece of paper upside down.
4. On the other half of the paper, I traced the letters made in step 2 or copied their lines. In doing so, I explained that I tried not to think about letters as such but only as drawing marks and that the best way to do this is to empty the mind and think about nothing but be aware if something unexpected comes into the mind or if feelings surface.
5. Finally, I turned the piece of paper back to its original position and looked at it, explaining that I observed the letters or let the image "speak back" while I paid attention to what I was thinking about and feeling.

John seemed keen to try out the method. He began with the word *LESTUR* Icel. (see Figure 8.5). Then he turned the paper upside down and drew the letterforms reversed. He drew the letters upside down as instructed but mirrored the letters from right to left. John did not say much while doing this. He then wished

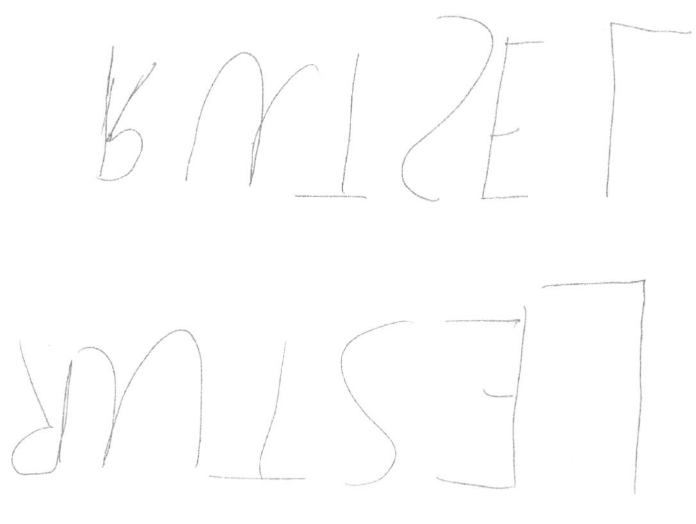

FIGURE 8.5

to draw/write his name in the same way. When he drew his name upside down, he played with the letters as if they were reflected in water.

Then he wanted to draw an image. While drawing (see Figure 8.6), John spontaneously explained: "I'm trying to draw a bridge that my great grandfather built . . . His name was also John. He was a famous bridge builder." On the left-hand side of the image, he wrote: "There is a big, deep river under my feet, and I stand on a footpath that is connected to many bars and a lot of concrete. The handrail rises ten metres into the air, 12 lamp posts stand on the concrete, and thick bars go into the river attached to the handrail, or bars and concrete. More than twelve-metre-high cliffs rise from the river, and only a few cars drive on the road within half an hour; most of them are big, and small islands only 20 metres long and high rise from the river" (English translation).

When he finished writing, he read out loud what he had written. In the story, everything is huge: the river, the bridge, the handrail, the cliffs and the cars crossing the bridge. I considered whether he was attempting to bridge or integrate his emotional and cognitive parts symbolised by the drawn bridge. The bridge in the drawing looks rather fragile, which may indicate that the integration had just begun and was not yet very stable.

After John had finished reading the text, I mirrored back by saying that it was a really big bridge. His reading was faster than in earlier sessions. He appeared satisfied when he said: "Now it is different to read. I'm less tired."

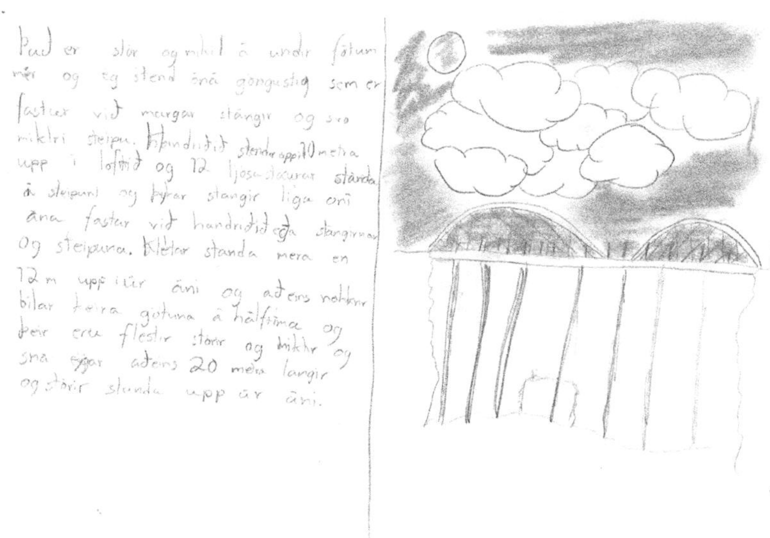

FIGURE 8.6 Memory drawing.

Results of the case study and grounded theory analysis

One of the main categories that emerged through the grounded theory analysis was the function of art-making, which includes memorising through drawing as one of its subcategories. The focus of the present writing is on the part of the grounded theory results that relate to memory drawing for the purpose of processing emotions relating to stress and/or trauma and memorising coursework through such drawing.

One way that emotional and cognitive functions are integrated into art therapy is when making the art and then verbalising its content. Further such integration takes place in other art therapy approaches, such as the ATTP method, when additional body movement is included in the art-making process through walking (Talwar, 2007). In AET, an additional integration between emotional and cognitive functions takes place when the intellectual, educational and cognitive coursework material is worked with while simultaneously working with therapeutic emotional aspects within one artwork.

An example of such integration is when John chose to draw the word *yfirbugaðir* Icel. ("overwhelmed" in English), which had to do with the spelling rule that he was studying. This is an educational approach, which at the same time may have been related to stress and/or trauma and being overwhelmed by too much emotional material emerging. There may also have been, to some degree, a shortage of containment and time available, which is a therapeutic perspective. He may have been overwhelmed by memorising and understanding the spelling rule itself, which may have been an echo or projection of his emotions regarding his difficult life experiences. When learning the spelling rule and making drawings out of the letters, further integration took place (see Figure 8.1), while the emotional content was still more prominent when making Figure 8.4 about Hilter's machine. An additional integration between the intellectual coursework learning and non-verbal functions, which can relate more to the emotional material, took place when John drew the lines of the letters upside down, focusing on the forms and lines of the letters while excluding the sound of the letters and the meaning of the word, which was then followed by the bridge drawing (see Figure 8.6). Thus, AET includes, in various ways, a dance between emotional art therapeutic work and coursework learning where intellectual and emotional processes are intertwined.

Twelve years after therapy ended, when John was 24 years old, a person who was interested in studying AET conducted an interview with him about his experience of the therapy. He said about his experience with the therapy: "I was taught in AET to apply the therapy as a concentrating and soothing method because when I was a child, I did not have the concentration to learn anything. I have also used the AET to learn mathematics and spelling. When spelling, I applied this method to remember words and pictures . . . Since then,

I have tended to draw words instead of writing letters . . . I still use the same method to remember the spelling of words . . . I also think that therapy helped me with social contact and self-esteem . . . I didn't see AET either as education or therapy, I just found it to be fun after school."

The intertwined emotional and intellectual qualities of AET shine through John's feedback 12 years after therapy ended. He emphasised the memorisation quality of his drawings. He also stated that he experienced increased concentration through the therapy, as well as mentioned its soothing quality which could relate to the emotional processing, containment and regulation that were offered to him through the therapeutic relationship, coursework learning and art-making, including memory drawing. Additionally, he mentioned an increase in self-esteem, which may have been a result of the therapy as he came into contact with himself through art-making and the therapeutic relationship, as well as being able to master his coursework learning. He also mentioned that the therapy was fun after school, which could relate to the way he was able to apply the playful quality of art-making to his emotional processing and coursework learning.

John's school grades and findings from psychological testing from before and after therapy were compared. Most of John's school grades improved following therapy. John's IQ score was 16 points higher after therapy. John's social skills also improved following the therapy, according to the results from the Child Behavior Checklist, which his mother completed. These findings indicate that the therapy helped John in his coursework learning and that it facilitated his well-being.

Discussion

Memory drawing for children who have experienced stress and/or trauma

From all the words John could have found in the dictionary that had "y" in them, he chose to draw about the content of the word *yfirbugaðir* Icel. ("overwhelmed" in English) when he was learning a spelling rule relating to when to write "y" or "i" in Icelandic (see Figure 8.1). John could have been working with his overwhelming feelings through the drawing, relating to the stress and/or trauma he had experienced regarding his parent's divorce, the illness and loss of his grandparents, the tiredness of his mother and missing his father, in addition to dealing with his specific learning difficulty.

John's mother may, at times, have been unable to contain the boy's feelings due to her own stress, trauma and/or tiredness. John made four containers out of letters when he drew Figure 8.1, which may have indicated that the treatment provided emotional containment for him through the therapeutic relationship and his memory drawing, which in turn might have facilitated his thinking and coursework learning. John appeared to be working with his emotions relating to care and containment as well as the stress and/or trauma he had experienced, in addition to simultaneously memorising a spelling rule and spelling of a word in therapy through making Figure 8.1.

Integrating coursework learning into art therapy was seen as part of managing and regulating feelings of vulnerability, which may stem from memories of trauma. The case study findings indicate that feelings of vulnerability can emerge and be processed through memory drawing. It was hypothesised that there was a link between John's specific learning difficulty and the emotions stemming from the difficulties he had experienced. At the time of language acquisition and when he started to learn to read and write at school, the people he was close to were either dealing with a variety of difficulties or they had left, and therefore they may have been to some degree unable to adequately contain the boy's emotions. Consequently, John may have felt overwhelmed by his feelings and lacked a space to think, which might partly explain his difficulty concentrating while learning to read and write.

The emotional processing and coursework learning came together in the memory drawing, such as when John was learning and memorising the spelling of the word "overwhelmed." In that way, through the memory drawing, he appeared to be processing emotions which related to the meaning of the word and his difficult experiences at the same time as he was learning the spelling of the word.

The case study vignettes presented in this chapter demonstrate the way in which memory drawing can be applied to integrate coursework learning, drawing and emotional processing. The findings of the study indicated that drawing was a productive way for the children to remember their coursework learning, such as when John remembered the spelling rule correctly (Figure 8.2 repeated) by thinking about the memory drawings he had made earlier (Figure 8.1). This was also supported by John's feedback, which he gave 12 years after therapy when he said that he found drawing helped him to memorise how to spell words and that he was still using the method, which he learnt in therapy, to memorise.

Limitations of the study

The findings of the present study indicate that the therapy worked well for John, which is the basis of a hypothesis that the method can be effective for other children who have experienced stress and/or trauma and deal with specific learning difficulties. The case study method was found to be useful to study in-depth the new AET method and the complex individual therapeutic and learning processes of each child. In addition, the grounded theory research methodology was found to be useful in building an initial theory of the AET method developed, including the formation of the concept and category "memory through drawing" and its connections to other parts of the theory (Óttarsdóttir, 2013). Although the research design was found to be useful for the purpose of developing AET at this early stage and for investigating how coursework, including memory drawing, can be included in art therapy, additional further studies could be conducted to study the function and effectiveness of the method more rigorously.

Implications for policy and practice

Increased knowledge within the school system about AET and its foundations, including art therapy methods and theories, is important for facilitating the integration of AET into education. It is also important for art therapists to have some knowledge about education when incorporating memory drawing into their practice.

One part of integrating memory drawing into education is thus a curriculum for art therapists working in schools. This particular curriculum and education would include information about findings from case studies, such as that reviewed in this chapter, which depicts the way in which drawing can be applied when memorising and learning coursework, along with the emotional work included. The curriculum comprises information about the way in which the processes that occur within AET are intertwined with regard to art-making, emotional processing, coursework learning and memorising. Education and curriculum, which refer to the research findings presented in this chapter, are an important part of creating a channel for incorporating the art therapeutically based AET into education.

Conclusion

Memory through drawing is a method developed and studied through the case study involving children who had experienced stress and/or trauma and had specific learning difficulties. Memory drawing is a concept included in the theory of AET, which emerged through the study and reveals a close connection between art therapy and coursework learning. The manner in which coursework learning can be integrated into art therapy was explored and demonstrated through the case studies, as shown in the vignettes presented in this chapter. These include Figure 8.1, where John made images out of letters, and Figure 8.4, in which he simultaneously processed his overwhelming feelings relating to stress and/or trauma while memorising a spelling rule and spelling of a specific word, *yfirbugaðir* Icel. ("overwhelmed" in English), which may be a consequence of the trauma. Further integration was facilitated when John drew letters upside down (see Figure 8.5) and when he made the bridge drawing (see Figure 8.6).

Providing an opportunity to process emotional material regarding memories relating to stress and/or trauma and simultaneously memorising coursework is made available in AET through art-making, including memory drawing and the therapeutic relationship. The containing quality of artwork made within the therapeutic relationship was found to have the potential to facilitate thinking and coursework learning. Also, integrating coursework into the therapy was found to have the potential to facilitate the regulation of overwhelming emotions caused by stress and/or trauma.

References

Abramovski, G., *et al.* (2019). Integrating art therapy in schools: a systematic literature review. *Studia Universitatis Babeş-Bolyai Psychologia-Paedagogia*, *64*(1), pp. 45–58. https://doi.org/10.24193/subbpsyped.2019.1.03.

Adoni-Kroyanker, M. *et al.* (2019). Practices and challenges in implementing art therapy in the school system. *International Journal of Art Therapy*, *24*(1), 40–49. https://doi.org/10.1080/17454832.2018.1536726.

Albert, R. (2010). Being both: An integrated model of art therapy and alternative art education. *Art Therapy*, *27*(2), 90–95. https://doi.org/10.1080/07421656.2010.10129713.

Appleton, V. (2001). Avenues of hope: art therapy and the resolution of trauma. *ARTherapy; Journal of the American Art Therapy Association*, *18*(1), 6–13. https://doi.org/10.1080/07421656.2001.10129454.

Avrahami, D. (2006). Visual art therapy's unique contribution in the treatment of post-traumatic stress disorders. *Journal of Trauma & Dissociation*, *6*(4), 5–38. https://doi.org/10.1300/J229v06n04_02.

Ayalon, A. (2021). The collaborative arts therapist-teacher model: theory and practice. In D. Regev and S. Snir (eds.), *Integrating Arts Therapies into Education a Collective Volume.* Oxford: Taylor & Francis Group.

Best, R. (2014). Educational psychotherapy: an approach to working with children whose learning is impeded by emotional problems. *Support for Learning*, *29*(3), 201–216. https://doi.org/10.1111/1467-9604.12058.

Bion, W. (1962a). The psycho-analytic study of thinking: ii. a theory of thinking. *International Journal of Psychoanalysis*, *10*(3), 306–310.

Bion, W. (1962b). *Learning from Experience*. London: Heinemann.

Case, C. (1990). Reflections and Shadows: an Exploration of the World of the Rejected Girl. In: C. Case and T. Dalley (eds.). *Working with children in art therapy*. London; New York: Routledge.

Case, C. (2003). Authenticity and survival working with children in chaos. *Inscape*, *8*(1), 17–28. https://doi.org/10.1080/17454830308414050.

Cohen, F.W. (1975). Introducing art therapy into a school system: some problems. *Art Psychotherapy*, *2*(2), 121–135. https://doi.org/10.1016/0090-9092(75)90014-9.

Dalley, T. (2000). Back to the future: thinking about theoretical developments in art therapy. In A. Gilroy and G. McNeilly (eds.), *The Changing Shape of Art Therapy*. London: Jessica Kingsley Publishers.

Deboys, R., Holttum, S. and Wright, K. (2016). Processes of change in school-based art therapy with children: a systematic qualitative study. *International Journal of Art Therapy*, *22*(3), 118–131. https://doi.org/10.1080/17454832.2016.1262882.

Dickson, C. (2015). Congruence of professional values: an exploration of the reciprocity between art teaching and art therapy. *ATOL: Art Therapy OnLine*, *6*(1), 1–16. https://doi.org/10.25602/GOLD.atol.v6i1.392

Dover, J. (2002). The child who cannot bear being taught. *Psychodynamic Practice*, *8*(3), 311–325.

Dover, J. (2003). Reaching and teaching the child who cannot trust. *The Resilient Child: How Coping and Resilience Promote and Develop the Capacity to Learn*. Norway: The Norwegian Educational Therapist Association, 164–171.

Eaton, L.G., Doherty, K.L. and Widrick, R.M. (2007). A review of research and methods used to establish art therapy as an effective treatment method for traumatized children. *The Arts in Psychotherapy*, *34*(3), 256–262. https://doi.org/10.1016/j.aip.2007.03.001.

Edwards, B. (2008). *The New Drawing on the Right Side of the Brain*. Expanded and updated ed. London: HarperCollins.

Edwards, D. (2004). *Art Therapy*. London: Sage Publications.

Fernandes, M.A., Wammes, J.D. and Meade, M.E. (2018). The Surprisingly powerful influence of drawing on memory. *Current Directions in Psychological Science*, *27*(5), 302–308. https://doi.org/10.1177/0963721418755385

Frydman, J.S., Hyman, S. and Caputo, S. (2022). Creative arts therapy in the United States school system: an integrative systematic review of empirically evaluated interventions from the past decade. *Psychology in the Schools*, *59*(3), 535–556. https://doi.org/10.1002/pits.22629.

Greenwood, A. (2002). The child who cannot bear to feel. *Psychodynamic Practice*, *8*(3), 295–310. https://doi.org/10.1080/1353333021000019015.

Harpazi, S. *et al.* (2020). Perceptions of art therapy in adolescent clients treated within the school system. *Frontiers in Psychology*, *11*, 518304. https://doi.org/10.3389/fpsyg.2020.518304.

Hass-Cohen, N., Bokoch, R. and Julia, M. (2022). A year later: the pain protocol study findings and memory reconsolidation factors. *The Arts in Psychotherapy*, *80*, 101949. https://doi.org/10.1016/j.aip.2022.101949.

Hass-Cohen, N. and Findlay, J.C. (2019). The art therapy relational neuroscience and memory reconsolidation four drawing protocol. *The Arts in Psychotherapy*, *63*, 51–59. https://doi.org/10.1016/j.aip.2019.03.002.

Herman, J.L. (2015) *Trauma and Recovery*. New York: BasicBooks.

Jalava, S.T., Wammes, J.D. and Cheng, K. (2023). Drawing your way to an A: Long-lasting improvements in classroom quiz performance following drawing. *Psychonomic Bulletin & Review* [Preprint]. https://doi.org/10.3758/s13423-023-02294-2.

Karp, C.L. and Butler, T.L. (1996). *Treatment Strategies for Abused Children: From Victim to Survivor*. Thousand Oaks: Sage Publications (Interpersonal violence).

Kozlowska, K. and Hanney, L. (2001). An art therapy group for children traumatized by parental violence and separation. *Clinical Child Psychology and Psychiatry*, *6*(1), 49–78.

Kramer, E. (1977). *Art Therapy in a Children's Community: A Study of the Function of Art Therapy in the Treatment Program of Wiltwyck School for Boys*. New York: Schocken Books.

Laub, D. and Podell, D. (1995). Art and trauma. *International Journal of Psychoanalysis*, *76*(5), 991–1005.

Malchiodi, C. (ed.). (2021). *Creative Interventions with Traumatized Children*. New York: Guilford.

Malchiodi, C.A. (1998). *Understanding Children's Drawings*. London: Jessica Kingsley Publishers.

Malchiodi, C.A. (ed.). (2012). *Handbook of Art Therapy*, 2nd edn. New York: Guilford Press.

McDonald, A. and Drey, N.S. (2017). Primary-school-based art therapy: a review of controlled studies. *International Journal of Art Therapy*, *23*(1), 1–12. https://doi.org/10.1080/17454832.2017.1338741.

McDonald, A. and Holttum, S. (2020). Primary-school-based art therapy: a mixed methods comparison study on children's classroom learning. *International Journal of Art Therapy*, *25*(3), 119–131. https://doi.org/10.1080/17454832.2020.1760906.

Meade, M.E., Ahmad, M. and Fernandes, M.A. (2020). Drawing pictures at encoding enhances memory in healthy older adults and in individuals with probable dementia. *Aging, Neuropsychology, and Cognition*, *27*(6), 880–901. https://doi.org/10.1080/13825585.2019.1700899.

Meade, M.E., Wammes, J.D. and Fernandes, M.A. (2018). Drawing as an encoding tool: memorial benefits in younger and older adults. *Experimental Aging Research*, *44*(5), 369–396. https://doi.org/10.1080/0361073X.2018.1521432.

Meade, M.E., Wammes, J.D. and Fernandes, M.A. (2019). Comparing the influence of doodling, drawing, and writing at encoding on memory. *Canadian Journal of Experimental Psychology/Revue canadienne de psychologie expérimentale*, *73*(1), 28–36. https://doi.org/10.1037/cep0000170.

Meyer, M.A. (1999). In exile from the body: creating a 'play room' in the 'waiting room'. In E.G. Levine and S.K. Levine (eds.), *Foundations of Expressive Art Therapy: Theoretical and Clinical Perspectives*. London: Jessica Kingsley Publishers.

Moula, Z. *et al.* (2020). A systematic review of child-focused outcomes and assessments of arts therapies delivered in primary mainstream schools. *Children and Youth Services Review*, *112*, 104928. Available at: https://doi.org/10.1016/j.childyouth.2020.104928

Moula, Z. *et al.* (2023). Child-focused outcome and process evaluation of a school-based art therapy intervention: a pilot randomised controlled study. *The Arts in Psychotherapy*, *86*, 102085. https://doi.org/10.1016/j.aip.2023.102085.

O'Brien, F. (2004). The making of mess in art therapy: attachment, trauma and the brain. *Inscape*, *9*(1), 2–13. https://doi.org/10.1080/02647140408405670.

Orr, P.P. (2007). Art therapy with children after a disaster: a content analysis. *The Arts in Psychotherapy*, *34*(4), 350–361. https://doi.org/10.1016/j.aip.2007.07.002.

Ottarsdottir, U. (2010a). Art therapy in education for children with specific learning difficulties who have experienced stress and/or trauma. In V. Karkou (ed.), *Arts Therapies in Schools: Research and Practice*. London: Jessica Kingsley Publishers.

Ottarsdottir, U. (2010b). Writing-images. *Art Therapy*, *27*(1), 32–39. https://doi.org/10.1080/07421656.2010.10129566.

Óttarsdóttir, U. (2013). Grunduð kenning og teiknaðar skýringarmyndir, In Sigríður Halldórsdóttir (ed.), *Handbók í aðferðafræði rannsókna*. Akureyri: University of Akureyri.

Ottarsdottir, U. (2018a). Art therapy to address emotional well-being of children who have experienced stress and/or trauma. In A. Zubala and V. Karkou (eds.), *Arts Therapies in the Treatment of Depression: International Research in the Arts Therapies*. Oxford: Routledge.

Ottarsdottir, U. (2018b). Processing emotions and memorising coursework through memory drawing. *Art Therapy Online*, *9*(1). https://doi.org/10.25602/GOLD.ATOL.V9I1.486

Ottarsdottir, U. (2019). Ethical concerns when applying drawing to promote memory: research conducted in Iceland. In A. Di Maria (ed.), *Exploring Ethical Dilemmas in Art Therapy: 50 Clinicians From 20 Countries Share Their Stories*. New York: Routledge/Taylor & Francis.

Ratnik, M. and Rüütel, E. (2019). The field of work of the school art therapist and its unique potential for the school support team. *Problems of Education in the 21st Century*, *77*(1), 142–155. https://doi.org/10.33225/pec/19.77.142.

Reddick, D. (2008). Working with the whole class in primary schools. In C. Case and T. Dalley (eds.), *Art Therapy with Children: From Infancy to Adolescence*. London and New York: Routledge.

Regev, D. (2022). A process-outcome study of school-based art therapy, *International Journal of Art Therapy*, *27*(1), 17–25. https://doi.org/10.1080/17454832.2021.1957960.

Regev, D. (2023). *Art Therapy with Special Education Students*. New York: Routledge.

Regev, D., Green-Orlovich, A. and Snir, S. (2015). Art therapy in schools: the therapist's perspective. *The Arts in Psychotherapy*, *45*, 47–55. https://doi.org/10.1016/j.aip.2015.07.004

Roberts, B.R.T. and Wammes, J.D. (2021). Drawing and memory: using visual production to alleviate concreteness effects. *Psychonomic Bulletin & Review*, *28*(1), 259–267. https://doi.org/10.3758/s13423-020-01804-w.

Rowe, C., *et al.* (2017). Evaluating art therapy to heal the effects of trauma among refugee youth: the burma art therapy program evaluation. *Health Promotion Practice*, *18*(1), 26–33. https://doi.org/10.1177/1524839915626413.

Rubin, J.A. (1999) *Art Therapy: An Introduction*. Philadelphia: Brunner/Mazel.

Schaverien, J. (1999). *The Revealing Image: Analytical Art Psychotherapy in Theory and Practice*. London, Philadelphia: Jessica Kingsley Publishers.

Schnitzer, G., Holttum, S. and Huet, V. (2021). A systematic literature review of the impact of art therapy upon post-traumatic stress disorder. *International Journal of Art Therapy*, *26*(4), 147–160. https://doi.org/10.1080/17454832.2021.1910719.

Strauss, A.L. and Corbin, J.M. (1998). *Basics of Qualitative Research: Techniques and Procedures for Developing Grounded Theory*, 2nd edn. Thousand Oaks: Sage Publications.

Talwar, S. (2007). Accessing traumatic memory through art making: an art therapy trauma protocol (ATTP). *The Arts in Psychotherapy*, *34*(1), 22–35. https://doi.org/10.1016/j.aip.2006.09.001.

Ugurlu, N., Akca, L. and Acarturk, C. (2016). An art therapy intervention for symptoms of post-traumatic stress, depression and anxiety among Syrian refugee children. *Vulnerable Children and Youth Studies*, *11*(2), 89–102. https://doi.org/10.1080/17450128.2016.1181288.

van der Kolk, B. (2007). The developmental impact of childhood trauma. In L.J. Kirmayer, R. Lemelson, and M. Barad (eds.), *Understanding Trauma: Integrating Biological, Clinical, and Cultural Perspectives*. Cambridge: Cambridge University Press. https://doi.org/10.1017/CBO9780511500008.

Wammes, J.D., Jonker, T.R. and Fernandes, M.A. (2019). Drawing improves memory: The importance of multimodal encoding context. *Cognition*, *191*, 103955. https://doi.org/10.1016/j.cognition.2019.04.024.

Wammes, J.D., Meade, M.E. and Fernandes, M.A. (2016). The drawing effect: Evidence for reliable and robust memory benefits in free recall. *The Quarterly Journal of Experimental Psychology*, *69*(9), 1752–1776. https://doi.org/10.1080/17470218.2015.1094494.

Wammes, J.D., Meade, M.E. and Fernandes, M.A. (2017). Learning terms and definitions: Drawing and the role of elaborative encoding. *Acta Psychologica*, *179*, 104–113. https://doi.org/10.1016/j.actpsy.2017.07.008.

Wammes, J.D., Meade, M.E. and Fernandes, M.A. (2018). Creating a recollection-based memory through drawing. *Journal of Experimental Psychology: Learning, Memory, and Cognition*, *44*(5), 734–751. https://doi.org/10.1037/xlm0000445.

Yin, R.K. (2014). *Case Study Research: Design and Methods*, 5th edn. Los Angeles: Sage.

9

THE LINGERING MEMORY OF WAR

A Duo-ethnographic Exploration on the Role of Dramatherapy in Revisiting and Honouring the Shadow of War in Refugee Women in Lebanon

Sara Sakhi, Farah Wardani, Lina H. Kreidie, Karima Anbar, and HH Sheikha Intisar Al Sabah

Abstract

The memories of war are unwanted visitors who often overstay their welcome long after the fighting is over. In this chapter, the authors revisit their experience with a group of refugee women in Lebanon who participated in a dramatherapy programme that took place in Shatila camp in 2019. The programme focused on the impact of war on women and resulted in a play entitled *Bayt Byout*. The context that surrounds refugee women is described, explaining the many social and personal ailments we witness in this community. We dive into the programme, describing how dramatherapy activities were used to reawaken the memories of war, and, later, how they were shared on a stage by those who held them.

Keywords: refugee women, Lebanon, dramatherapy, war, trauma

Abstract in Arabic

ذكريات الحرب هي زائر غير مرحب به، فهي غالبا ما تبقى لفترة طويلة بعد انتهاء الحرب . في هذا الفصل ، يعيد المؤلفون النظر في تجربتهم مع مجموعة من النساء اللاجئات في لبنان اللاتي شاركن في برنامج العلاج بالدراما الذي أقيم في مخيم شاتيلا في عام 2019. ركز البرنامج على تأثير الحرب على النساء و أسفر عن مسرحية بعنوان "بيت بيوت." يتم وصف الحالة التي تحيط باللاجئات ، و التي تفسر لاحقا العديد من الصعوبات الاجتماعية و الشخصية التي نشهدها في هذا المجتمع. نتعمق في هذا البرنامج ، و اصفين كيف تم استخدام أنشطة العلاج بالدراما لإعادة إحياء ذكريات الحرب ، و ثم بعد ذلك ، كيف تمت مشاركتها ببلاغة من قبل النساء اللواتي مررن بها على خشبة المسرح

DOI: 10.4324/9781032663944-9

Introduction

When considering how we can contribute to the richness of the world of creative art therapies research, we found our collective experiences of working with war-affected women to be deeply insightful. Since 2018, the Intisar Foundation has put forth efforts to bridge the gaps in mental health for the millions of women affected by war in the Arab world. Drama seemed to be an ideal approach to address the festering invisible wounds left behind and to gently unearth memories buried deep within individual and collective minds. For this chapter, the practising facilitator of dramatherapy, Farah Wardani, and the researcher, Sara Sakhi, sat down for a conversation and an interview. They discussed how the memory of war exists in a deafening silence that permeates refugee camps and neighbourhoods in Lebanon and how society had macroscopically decided to shun the topic of war and ignore all its ramifications. Both Farah, as the facilitator, and Sara, as the observer, reflected on the women that walked into the dramatherapy sessions heavily laden with fear, pain and loneliness, and how the sessions opened a sacred space for revisiting and revising the past. Finally, they examined their own memories of the inner workings of dramatherapy and the processes they witnessed in one programme held in 2019 with 21 predominantly Syrian refugee women in Shatila refugee camp.

This chapter is a reflexive duo-ethnographic examination of these experiences. The methodological approach included an interview, past session and programme reports, and a playscript written in collaboration with the participants. The authors opted to combine all this information into a comprehensive chapter that informs the reader while drawing from different retrospective sources that were compiled and threaded together through reflections and memories. The chapter aims to draw a complete picture of dramatherapy's role in honouring the memories of war in women whose entire identities have become defined by their past. In addition, the chapter sheds light not only on the programme and the women but also on the contexts that surround them. Dramatherapy is an approach that, as we observed, could transport the participants to any space and at any time. It offered a sense of community that is lacking in their daily lives and a chance to be seen and validated by their peers. Their experiences and memories are normalised and concretised by the others, who have themselves lived through the horrors of war.

Part I: Refugee women in Lebanon and the countless struggles for survival

The memories of war linger in the narrow pathways, overcrowded homes and busy streets of Beirut. Lebanon is a small Mediterranean country with a tumultuous history. In its brief history leading up to its independence, Lebanon has witnessed French colonialism, religious and political chasms, civil wars, military occupations and several waves of refugees seeking safety on its land. Lebanon retains the highest ratio of refugees per capita, and its local population has witnessed myriad wars and armed conflicts. Over 1.5 million Syrian refugees have fled to Lebanon since 2011, and nearly half a million Palestinian refugees have resided there in protracted exile since 1948 (Kiwan, 2019). The total population hovers around 5.5 million as of 2021 (World Bank, 2021), making the total refugee population upwards of 35%.

More recently, a domino effect of crises has plagued the country, with 2019 protests triggering the resignation of the government, the severe devaluation of the Lebanese pound against the US Dollar and crumbling economic and social structures (Manduchi, 2021). The situation has reached most corners of the country, but it is especially pronounced in the refugee camps and refugee-dense neighbourhoods. In Shatila camp, located in southern Beirut, illegal construction crowds out the sun. Utilities are secured privately through electricity mafias or are completely non-existent. Many children drop out or never enrol in school, opting instead to work menial jobs to support their families with meagre pay. Within this settlement, war, displacement, racism, bigotry, poverty, hopelessness and violence have enmeshed themselves in the fabric of living.

With the ongoing crises, refugees seem to have no end in sight for their suffering. The trauma of war, loss and displacement has been overshadowed by the daily struggle to survive, the rejected asylum applications to western European states and the fears of mounting bills and cost of living. The topic of war is sensitive and difficult to approach during turbulent times. Often, focus and energy are expended on the struggle to maintain what little well-being and control one has, rather than addressing past events. The accepted narrative of keeping up with daily life has blunted grief and pushed forward the façade of resilience. However, as observed time and again in the realm of psychology, unaddressed trauma re-emerges.

The memories of war maintain their prominent place within most refugees, expressing themselves with unusually high levels of depression (Naal, *et al.*, 2021), post-traumatic stress disorder (PTSD) (Haddad Kreidie, *et al.*, 2016), and inter-generational trauma (Kelstrup and Carlsson, 2022). The effects seep into daily life, beyond diagnosable symptomology and into the social interactions and commonly accepted principles of behaviour. Collectively experienced traumatic events live on, reshaping individual and collective identities with narratives of victimhood (Hirschberger, 2018) and prompting negative social dynamics like fragmentation (Theisen-Womersley, 2021).

Part II: The loneliness of crowds

War challenges many of the concepts we dearly hold on to and forces us to realise our limitations at the barrel of a gun. A person can lose everything they cherish, their family, their homes and their homeland. But, more importantly, control and autonomy are lost. War accentuates our weaknesses and the fragility of comfort we build in our lives. Most refugees cannot face this reality, although they have already witnessed it. Accepting it and reconciling with it is a new challenge on top of surviving in a hostile environment.

Their past lingers, as many have testified during dramatherapy sessions, as nightmares and emotional outbursts that provide temporary emotional relief. Their once-injured limbs flare up with pain when they are confronted with a new problem. Their voices hesitate when they speak about the past, it is so far bygone and so abstract now. Women who sent their children to school at seven in the morning, tended to their vast gardens until noon and enjoyed evening tea with friends are now sharing a room deprived of sunlight with another family. Their well-established identities become lost as they navigate the social complexities of being a refugee and having lost the jobs, people and possessions that helped define them (Douglas, 2010). Legal and socio-economic discrimination reduce opportunities for decent work and living (Chit and Nayel, 2013; OHCHR, 2021), whereas racism and social discrimination prevent integration and enjoying a sense of safety in Lebanon (El Daoi, 2020).

Despite living in some of the most densely populated areas in Lebanon, with Shatila camp holding up to 20,000 residents in a one square kilometre area (Puig, 2020), refugee women can live incredibly lonely lives. Many dysfunctional behaviours and attitudes result from the compounded and continued trauma of living as a refugee in Lebanon. The issue is worsened not only by the barriers to accessing mental health resources but the social complexities that arise because of these traumas and the collective coping mechanism of ignoring the past and hiding its wounds.

"Check-in" activities are used at the beginning of the sessions to gauge the participants' current emotional state. In the initial stages of the programme, when we ask the participants "How are you today?" the answers are usually, "Thank God," "Still Living," or "Still managing." These responses are indicative of avoidance, one of the symptom clusters of PTSD. Avoidance is defined as actively evading the topics, places or experiences that remind a person of their traumatic experience, by emotional numbing, and gaps in memory relating to the traumatic event (Norris and Aroian, 2008). Because trauma is never experienced in a vacuum, many will look towards others to gauge their reactions and coping mechanisms and derive a normative behavioural pattern. While avoidance may temporarily blunt emotional responses and provide short-term comfort, in the long term it often leads to maladaptive behaviours and reduces the likelihood of seeking mental health support (Bryant, 2022).

The refugee population in Lebanon is often lauded for its resilience despite all the hardships it has faced (Dionigi, 2016; Popham, *et al.*, 2022). In the simplest terms, psychological resilience is defined as the ability to cope in the face of difficulty and return to the pre-crisis levels of well-being (Southwick, *et al.*, 2014). Resilience is considered a positive reaction to the various difficulties of life, and the normative levels of resilience and vulnerability are often defined by professionals rather than those who experienced the struggles themselves (Schwarz, 2018). However, it is important to note that resilience may hide emotional avoidance and repressive coping. For many refugee women, there is never a place or time to grieve their losses or to acknowledge their pain. Instead, the pressures of survival and having basic needs met are always prioritised. Internalised ideals to remain resilient completely disregard the justifiable emotional reactions that would arise when an entire group has been deprived of all hope. The concept of patience in the face of adversity is a popular tenet in Islamic belief (Rusdi, 2016) and Christianity (Schnitker, *et al.*, 2017), which are the dominant religious philosophies that inform cultural beliefs in the region. As most of these refugee women are practising Muslims, there is a chance their faith and surroundings encourage them to remain patient. While patience has many benefits, the long drawn-out struggles of an oppressed group with little hope in its future cannot be overlooked or overcome easily. The resilience of refugee women in Lebanon is a resilience of hopelessness, not of hope.

The refugees in Lebanon also live alongside other war survivors in the local population. Many Lebanese people have witnessed one or more violent episodes or periods of armed conflict, making Lebanon a country where little space for healing or progress exists. Conversations or personal disclosure about war, trauma and loss are not tolerated when everyone else is burdened by their own stories. If one woman lost her son, the neighbour lost all her children. If one family can barely afford bread, the family down the street regularly eats from the garbage pails. And if one community cannot cope with their past, the entire country struggles with painful memories. Thus, many of the women we work with often cite others' suffering as a point of reference to their own. The line of reasoning often follows this sequence:
-I witnessed a horrible event.

- I feel distressed.
- My behaviour has changed for the worse.
- My neighbour witnessed a more horrible event.
- My neighbour appears to function properly.
- I must function properly.

This reasoning reverberates across communities and leads to the individual losing ownership over their narrative. The personal story of war melts and solidifies into a coagulated mass that lacks definition. Everyone has a horrible story to share, and one person sharing it is seen as an attention-seeker or a weakling. Nonetheless, even if hundreds of millions experienced the same event, the personal story still carries its weight and significance. It still holds an impact on the individual, and thereby collective, well-being.

Hence, approaching the topic of war is a difficult exercise in balance. On the one hand, practitioners must aim to create a welcoming and safe space to encourage participants to slowly unravel the layers of avoidance. On the other hand, meticulous care must be taken to avoid triggering a flood of re-traumatisation before strong enough foundations have been established. The participants should be made to realise that they are, in fact, entitled to their grief. And despite everything their past and circumstances have taught them, they are entitled to experience and express their emotions in a way that is right for them.

Part III: Dramatherapy in refugee camps

Traditional psychological interventions in Lebanon often follow procedures that have originated from and developed in the global north. Scientific literature in most fields, too, is often written in the English language (Hamel, 2007). This especially poses a challenge for non-Western countries in fields where cultural subtleties take precedence, like psychology. More importantly, the limitations of talking therapy do not allow it to address all the manifestations of war-related trauma. Notably, research on civilians impacted by war has shown a strong link to somatic symptoms, or physically expressed signs of distress (Sack, *et al.*, 2007), with women having higher levels of somatisation (Morina, *et al.*, 2018). We often see women seeking out general physicians to help them cope with their sleeping issues, headaches and chronic fatigue.

The doctors are usually content to ignore the root psychological issue, which is too sensitive and humanising to address in the clinical setting. Instead, we see women of different age groups on multiple prescriptions that numb their pain, sometimes taking anti-depressants prescribed by a family doctor who neglects to inform them of the real purpose of such medicines and does not refer them to further professionals. Many primary care physicians in Lebanon prescribe psychoactive drugs to patients without fully informing them of the prognosis and side effects (El Zahran, *et al.*, 2023). This gap in the access and provision of long-term mental health care underlines the need for alternative care.

The urgent need for mental health care for refugees in Lebanon is met with many barriers, some systemic and others cultural. The stigma of clinical and medicalised mental health care is significant in both the local and refugee communities, preventing many in need of support from seeking it (El Chammay, 2016). The expensive and privatised Lebanese healthcare system prevents refugees and low socio-economic status Lebanese nationals from even considering their options, as over 90% of Syrian refugees live in extreme poverty (UNHCR, 2022) and 82% of Lebanese households live in multidimensional poverty (ESCWA, 2021). Further, the lack of free and local programmes forces many to travel outside their areas to find professionals. Hence, many live with untreated and debilitating mental health issues that interfere with their daily lives and ability to live comfortably.

Since 2018, the Intisar Foundation has facilitated dramatherapy programmes for women impacted by war in Lebanon and Jordan with the goal of alleviating psychological distress, building resilience and creating bottom-up social change. The unconventional approach of dramatherapy offers a solution for the many barriers refugee women face in accessing mental health resources. Firstly, by presenting the programmes as a cultural activity rather than a medical or psychological intervention, it is able to circumvent the stigma associated with mental health care. Secondly, the programmes are offered free of charge and implemented inside camps and neighbourhoods with the support of local entities and NGOs. Thus, the participants would often feel safer and more incentivised to attend dramatherapy programmes as opposed to entering a mental health clinic or psychiatric hospital. Furthermore, the stigma of seeking mental health support does not apply in programmes like dramatherapy, which can be easily justified to husbands and neighbours as a light-hearted group cultural activity. Implementing the programmes in local centres within the camps and impacted areas builds further trust in those in the local community who are often distrustful of foreign NGOs.

Despite the many barriers preventing access to mental health support, we ensure our programmes provide the best possible conditions to encourage enrolment, attendance and retention. Hence, to meet the needs of the participants, we take into consideration the duration, location and even the time of day and day of the week. In addition to logistical conveniences for the participants, such as the travel distance and familiarity with the location, the programmes are implemented in these areas to help the local community develop and grow. By working within the community for prolonged periods of time, we ensure our programmes not only target individual well-being and mental health but also improve social cohesion and community resilience. Therefore, the programmes are always implemented inside areas with a high density of refugees, such as refugee camps or neighbourhoods with high levels of resettlement.

We had to consider many logistical barriers in addition to cultural and economic ones while planning our programmes. Most of the participants are married mothers with children who attend specialised schools that hold classes in the afternoons. In general, most refugee women do not have a conventional 9-to-5 job and usually bear all the household duties. Hence, morning timeslots are preferred, when their children are still safely at home and they do not need to prepare any housework. Following this logic, while most adult programmes might choose an evening time slot, we work in the mornings when the women can get out of the house and have time for themselves. The sessions always take place in the same place and on the same day of the week, building a sense of routine for the participants. They are thus able to plan their week ahead, scheduling any appointments or chores around the sessions.

Part IV: Methodology

For this chapter, a duo-ethnographic approach was used. Farah and Sara worked together for over three years under the Intisar Foundation, both experiencing the same programmes from different perspectives. Duo-ethnography is a qualitative approach that provides an understanding of one phenomenon experienced by two or more individuals (Noris, *et al.*, 2012). This approach was used to allow both of us to reflect on our experiences in tandem. The first step was to discuss and reflect on which groups/programmes we should focus on to convey our topic of "honouring the memory of war." After we decided on the 2019 programme, we sat down for a long, audio-recorded interview and discussion guided by a series of questions we thought would be relevant to provide the necessary insights. Following the interview, the audio was transcribed. The transcript allowed us to pinpoint the most prominent themes and commence writing, with regular revisions and discussions on the content with support from our co-authors. At many points, we needed guidance and reflection, as different vantage points facilitated broadening perspectives and new insights into events we had taken for granted.

Before laying out the final structure, we highlighted a series of topics necessary as foundational information to help the reader understand the full context of the population, the history and modern situation in Lebanon, and why the approach of dramatherapy has been used. Hence, we wrote a comprehensive literature review that provides insights into the sphere of conditions that led up to the 2019 programme and beyond. Finally, we supplemented our discussions with pre-existing material, examining our backlog of session reports, scripts and notes from 2019 to provide concrete examples, as seen below in the example session activities and vignettes.

Participants

The programme was implemented with support from Basmeh & Zeitooneh (2023) in Shatila camp, a relief and development organisation for Syrian refugees, which provided the facilities and outreach. The participants were recruited through social workers at the centre, who had a long-established relationship with the community, as well as some participants who heard about the programmes through word of mouth. A total of 21 participants joined the programmes which started in March 2019 and ended in July 2019. The participants' average age was 43 years, with most being homemakers, apart from five employed in various sectors. All were women, most were married with children, and all but one were of Syrian origin, with the outlier being a Lebanese national who lived in Syria for 20 years.

Session design

The programme was designed to approach social and personal issues using creativity, embodiment and shared experiences. Although the sessions remain amendable, and the phases overlap or change duration depending on the needs of the groups and individuals within them, the general structure of the five-phase model originated by Renée Emunah (2019) is followed in the programme. While the programme aimed to alleviate emotional distress, develop skills and create a bond among the participants, larger issues for this community could not realistically be addressed throughout. For example, the lack of access to basic needs, extreme poverty, and the lack of legal or social stability are issues that continue to plague the refugee community in Lebanon. While the programme may have provided some level of reduction in the stress and loneliness often felt in Shatila camp, it could not address serious psychiatric issues which continue to exist due to the stigma and barriers surrounding mental health access. The following section outlines how the five-phase model is adapted to fit the context of the camp and also produce a play based on the personal stories of the participants, of which a selection is shared in the vignettes below.

Dramatic play and scene work

The programmes aim first to establish a sense of trust and openness to new experiences related to theatre and movement. As trust is often difficult to establish in groups that have experienced marginalisation, activities start out fairly simple, requiring a physical gesture instead of speaking, to encourage self-disclosure. Examples include "Step Inside" (Fox, 2010), where the facilitator asks the participants to step forwards if the statement applies to them. The first phase is also rich with preliminary theatre activities that work on developing group dynamics and exploration of embodiment. The use of the body is heavily emphasised as a tool for both expression and awareness. This exercise starts out simply enough, "step forwards if you have a sister," "step forwards if you made lunch yesterday." As comfort levels even out, the participants are pushed to reveal more personal aspects of themselves. "Step forwards if you lost someone you love in the war" is often used to offer a space to recognise both loss and identity. Similarly, a compact activity like "Rose and Thorn" (Fox, 2010) provides quick and brief insights into each participant's life. This activity consists of a reflection on the most prominently present positives and negatives in each participant's life, with the positive being the rose and the negatives being the thorn. For example, one participant may say "My rose is my daughter, my thorn is the poverty we live in."

In "Image Theatre" (Boal, 1995), the participants form groups, embody an image they want to express and create a living picture in front of the group.

The group is then asked to analyse and interpret the picture. Such an activity works on all the above-mentioned elements, adding the element of being seen, witnessed and appreciated by the group. In an exercise entitled "Picture Theatre," we see groups of women barely familiar with each other beginning to form sculptures reminiscent of war, life before displacement and everyday life. When the discussion or reflection takes place after the activity, the participants reveal why they chose to portray such a sculpture.

"Picture Theatre" was used in the early stages of the programme. One group depicted children playing while a rocket flew towards them. This picture sparked many recollections of the war, as many had lived through it, escaping rockets launched at their villages and homes. Here, the memory of war is embodied and seen, prompting a sense of cohesion as the defining feature of the group is their war experience. A truth often unspoken surfaces through the silent sculpture the participants had come up with on their own. The reflection following the activity sees the participants growing more comfortable with self-disclosure and sharing personal memories.

Role play and culminating enactments

As the group members become more familiar with each other and a sense of safety prevails, more inquisitive and probing activities start to take place. A perfect example is "Life map," where a section of the room acts as a stage, and the group members act as an audience. One by one, the participants approach the stage, disclosing what they deem as the most important stages of their lives. Few instructions precede this activity, as participants are encouraged to discover their life events at a pace that suits them. The most important aspect of working in a group within dramatherapy, as observed through our experiences, is the impact one participant's openness has on the rest. When even one participant is brave enough to share a deeply private aspect of herself, the self-consciousness of others disappears gradually. They are emboldened by others' boldness. "Life Map" is usually situated around the fifth or sixth session, where the programme has set enough foundational work to slowly push towards deeper subjects.

In "Life Map," many women start to explore the war and its implications on their lives. "Here," a participant would say as she steps forwards on her imagined map, "we started to hear aerial bombing nearly every day, my children stopped going to school." Another step in a different direction: "We packed the necessary clothes and medicines, leaving behind my beloved vases and curtains, and left the house at two in the morning." Another step, "We crossed the border, thinking it would only be a few weeks, here we are seven years later." This activity provides both the space and witnesses needed to divulge such painful memories. The audience facing the participant is attentive and empathetic of her experience, many having been through similar events themselves. This activity is divided across several sessions, allowing the participants to take their time in exploring their first solo experience on a stage. This ensures, also, that the sessions can hold several activities for the rituals, warming up and releasing tension.

Imagination is often utilised throughout the programme to aid in retrieving memories. One of the hallmarks of group work is how one activity can evoke different reactions in different participants. For example, a commonly used activity in these phases revolves around the use of imagination to suspend time and space, a feat difficult to achieve outside the realm of drama. A walking, guided meditation is aided by gentle music, allowing the participants to imagine themselves in a new city. They are prompted to take in the smells of coffee and flowers on a new street and gently pushed to imagine their bodies draped in elegant and colourful clothing, the cobblestone roads beneath their feet. As their imagination deepens, their backs straighten and their feet lift with more grace off the ground. "Is that music you're hearing?" the facilitator softly announces, adding a new dimension to their experience. "Explore the space around you with your body, sway to the rhythm." Dancing now, the participants end the activity smiling and exchanging eye contact, a rare sight in the camp.

Soon, when the group reflects on the activity, they reveal a trip back in time. The Aleppo streets bursting with jasmine shrubs and the dizzying sweetness of their scent, the bumpiness of the road they travelled every day on their way to the market. How these little pleasures were taken from them, replaced now by dangerous electric wires hanging low above heads in the camp and puddles of dirty water that keep their eyes glued to the ground as they walk. Music and dance are a delicacy enjoyed only on special occasions, if they ever arise. Many participants share that they have not danced in years for various reasons. It could be the simple lack of personal space in their cramped homes or the heaviness carried in their bodies. This activity is followed by "Well of Secrets," where the memories and hopes are verbalised and actualised into the world, witnessed by others then promptly thrown into a collectively imagined well that holds all their secrets. This activity was developed by Farah Wardani, who saw a need in the populations she has worked with to openly share their secrets in a way that guarantees they are safely "discarded" and thereby never discussed again unless the person sharing invites the gesture.

The topic of war comes up organically as the programme progresses; although it is a fundamental theme in the construction of their identities and histories, we see a near-total absence of its mention in daily life. When an activity like "Mirror Monologue" is used, the participants are asked to contemplate their facial features in a small handheld mirror and share out loud their thoughts about their faces. Many women start by expressing how long it has been since they looked in a mirror and that their faces have changed compared to how they pictured them. Slowly, they reveal more and more about themselves, the dark circles under their eyes signify sleepless nights spent in cramped rooms, laying on thin mattresses in the unforgiving heat of Beirut. Each wrinkle tells a different story of loss, pain and exile. This activity was developed by Farah Wardani, who was inspired by feminine rituals related to self-care and speech therapy techniques in which a mirror is used to help practise mouth movements (Hamerlińska and Kieczmer, 2020).

Towards the last quarter of the programme, more complex and investigative activities take place. One example is the game of projection that uses small toys or figurines (Jones, 2007) to bring forth ideas hiding in the back of the mind. This activity utilises Jungian archetypes to facilitate a therapeutic process. Following a relaxing meditative activity, a collection of small toys or figurines is placed in the centre of the room, the participants are asked to walk around, pick up an item, examine it and place it back. This is repeated a few times until each participant has found an item that speaks to them. They are then asked to sit down in an audience formation and talk about why they chose this particular item. In this activity, many memories are recalled as the tangibility and absurdity of the item prompts a unique connection. Aeroplanes and ships are often picked first. Perhaps they represent the wish to flee Lebanon. A small doll may represent a grandmother's gift that has been long lost in the wreckage and will never be held again. A small duck may be a reminder of the pond and animals that lived close to their previous home. A pink shoe perhaps reminds one participant of her granddaughter who was born back in Syria.

Dramatic ritual

While not all the groups we worked with had a chance to do a performance, especially after the Covid-19 pandemic prevented larger gatherings, one group had a chance to perform their play in front of an audience. The play was entitled *Bayt Byout*, a transliteration of an Arabic term used to describe a childhood game of playing house. The performance was a vignette play centred on the themes of women, forced displacement and living as a refugee. The various segments were written and imagined by the participants, who hung their dreams and most vulnerable moments against a black backdrop. Throughout the progression of the programme, the facilitator noted important moments of personal disclosure that later became these vignettes. The vignettes in this chapter were shared publicly during the performance and informed consent to share, republish and reuse visual and written materials was obtained from the participants before the performance. The participants were encouraged to share the themes they wanted to explore in the play, and the scenes were created collaboratively and sewn together using props, light and music. Their stories explored themes of dispossession and loss, the inability to grieve their loss and the medicalisation of justified grief and emotional turmoil that ignores the larger picture. And finally, the hope is portrayed that can grow from even the most strenuous circumstances.

Vignette #14

A single ray of light spotlights a woman standing among various items on the ground.

> *Lebanon belongs to us; it belongs to the Syrians who escaped empty-handed. It is the crowded camps brimming with poverty, the dirty water we shower with, the exposed electric wiring hanging loosely, and the children walking barefoot amid rainy winter days. This is our Lebanon.*
>
> *I came across a graveyard in Shatila full of dead people, who may have met the dead we left behind on the streets of Syria in the afterlife. We were not able to cry for forty days; we could not honour them or grieve them. I would sit crying by a grave, cleansing the darkness and fear from my heart. One day the attendant noticed me and told me, "You are breaking my heart, every day I see you here crying at this grave, I started washing it every day in preparation for your visits. How are you related to him?"*
>
> *"I am not related to him, I am not related to any of them. I am grieving the people I never had a chance to grieve, I am mourning my house, my homeland, myself."*
>
> *The way he looked at me made me understand I was not welcomed there anymore. Even the graveyards had no place for us.*

She bends down, rummaging through the items around her and picking up a stone and a fabric doll.

> *All I have is a brick and a doll that I unearthed from the rubble of my destroyed home. I did not keep the brick to bash the heads of those who destroyed it, I kept it to retain a smell, a memory, a thing of my own in this world. Today, I own nothing in this world but this brick.*

Vignette #15

The stage is dark, and the sounds of clocks ticking are coupled with the sounds of bombs falling and people screaming. A woman is illuminated, her eyes search around as she anxiously starts her monologue.

> *The hour of war is upon us, and time starts to slow down, it never passes or ends. War is so far now, but its spectre haunts me. My children are safe, but I feel, no, I know, death is inching closer. Disease is inching closer. Depression is already here.*

She slightly changes her tone.

> *What do you mean by depression!? Do you think I'm crazy?*

She addresses two imaginary people on stage.

> *[Husband's name], [sister's name], what are you talking about? I am afraid, but my fear is justified, my madness is justified. I am dying on a daily basis. People are dying on a daily basis. I am not able to eat, drink, or sleep. Many people do not have anything to eat or drink, many have nowhere to sleep. I do not want to be medicated! I want the war to end! I am the broken, sad, depressed Syria that is no longer able to continue.*

She pauses and stands tall, becoming more composed.

> *They told me they will never leave me behind, so I took the medicine. I am better now, no longer depressed. But my beloved country is still depressed, and we have not found her a remedy.*

Vignette #20

A woman walks on stage, singing an Arabic song about the theatre. She is wearing a bright floral pink skirt, symbolising her inner child. She approaches a swing made of jute rope and a wooden board seat. She sits on the swing, swinging gently and starts her monologue.

> *I am not playing by myself; I am playing with my baby daughter. I am a mother, not a child, but I am 13 years old. My dream was to act, stand on stage, become a star, and go far in life. But he did not let me, he forced me to get married and forced me into this life. He deprived me of my life. He was such a despot, that only the war freed me from him. Yes, the war was the best thing to ever happen to me. It gave me freedom! My daughter was able to play, study, grow up, and write her own stage plays. My son is fulfilling his dreams of being a photographer. They are fulfilling the dreams I never could. Today I am avenging the little Syrian girl who rehearsed for a school play and was not allowed to perform in it. Today, I rehearsed, and I am performing on a stage, and I am living my dream! I am in front of an audience, who will see me, listen to me, and applaud my performance. I am Free! Free! Free!*

Conclusion

In this chapter, we revisited our experience with one group of Syrian refugee women who participated in a dramatherapy programme in 2019 and created a play about their life stories. The complexity of their memories and trauma was compounded by the inhospitable environment which left little room for healing. In Lebanon, the worsening economic situation, social stigma and lack of services made accessing mental health care a difficult feat, promoting the need for alternative solutions.

We found dramatherapy to be a suitable approach to not only alleviate emotional distress but also to share the participants' stories with the world. The creative expression and safety in numbers of the group setting allowed the participants to explore their past and future hopes. We examined our memories of the programme using reflexive duo-ethnography and existing documentation from the programme to write this chapter. This chapter provides an overview of the implementation and session design, showcasing a glimpse of the conclusion of this project through selected vignettes.

While the approach of dramatherapy cannot erase the past, we honoured the women's pasts and lived experiences. Our own memories of the project live on, as they do in the memories of the participants. The women we have worked with, and their stories, leave impressions on us that can never be forgotten or erased.

References

Basmeh and Zeitooneh. (2023). Shatila. Basmeh & Zeitooneh. Available at: https://www.basmeh-zeitooneh.org/our-locations/shatila

Boal, A. (1995). *The Rainbow of Desire: The Boal Method of Theatre and Therapy*. London and New York: Routledge.

Bryant, R.A. (2022). Post-traumatic stress disorder as moderator of other mental health conditions. *World Psychiatry, 21*(2), 310–311. https://doi.org/10.1002/wps.20975.

Chit, B. and Nayel, M.A. (2013). Understanding racism against Syrian refugees in Lebanon. *Civil Society Knowledge Centre*, 1(1). doi:https://doi.org/10.28943/cskc.002.10001.

Dionigi, F. (2016). *The Syrian Refugee Crisis in Lebanon: State Fragility and Social Resilience*. London: LSE Middle East Centre.

Douglas, A. (2010). Identities in transition: living as an asylum seeker. *Advances in Psychiatric Treatment, 16*(4), 238–244. https://doi.org/10.1192/apt.bp.108.006080.

El Chammay, R. (2016). Reforming mental health in Lebanon amid refugee crises. *Bulletin of the World Health Organization, 94*(8), 564–565. https://doi.org/10.2471/blt.16.030816.

El Daoi, R. (2020). Discrimination is part of our everyday lives. [online] *NRC*. Available at: https://www.nrc.no/perspectives/2020/discrimination-is-part-of-our-everyday-lives/ (accessed March 20, 2023).

El Zahran, T., Al Hassan, S., Khalifeh, M., Aboukhater, D., Hammoud, L., Al Hariri, M. and Kazzi, Z. (2023). Melitracen and flupentixol (deanxit) use disorder in Lebanon. *Heliyon, 9*(5), e15847. https://doi.org/10.1016/j.heliyon.2023.e15847.

Emunah, R. (2019). *Acting For Real*. Oxford: Routledge.

ESCWA. (2021). *Painful reality and uncertain prospects Poverty in Lebanon Multidimensional poverty* [online]. Geneva: UN ESCWA. Available at: https://www.unescwa.org/sites/default/files/news/docs/21-00634-_multidimentional_poverty_in_lebanon_-policy_brief_-_en.pdf (accessed March 13, 2023).

Fox, H. (2010). *Zoomy Zoomy: Improv Games and Exercises for Groups*. New Paltz, NY: Tusitala Publishing.

Haddad Kreidie, L., Kreidie, M. and Atassi, H. (2016). Living with ongoing political trauma: the prevalence and impact of PTSD among Syrian refugees. *Journal of Psychology Research, 6*(10). https://doi.org/10.17265/2159-5542/2016.10.005.

Hamel, R.E. (2007). The dominance of English in the international scientific periodical literature and the future of language use in science. *AILA Review*, *20*(1), 53–71. https://doi.org/10.1075/aila.20.06ham.

Hamerlińska, A. and Kieczmer, J. (2020). The use of the mirror in speech therapy. *Interdyscyplinarne Konteksty Pedagogiki Specjalnej*, *30*. https://doi.org/10.14746/ikps.2020.30.14.

Harvey, M.R. (1996). An ecological view of psychological trauma and trauma recovery. *Journal of Traumatic Stress*, *9*(1).

Hirschberger, G. (2018). Collective Trauma and the Social Construction of Meaning. *Frontiers in Psychology*, *9*(1441). https://doi.org/10.3389/fpsyg.2018.01441

Jones, P. (2007). *Drama as Therapy: Theory, Practice and Research*, 2nd edn. New York: Routledge.

Kelstrup, L. and Carlsson, J. (2022). Trauma-affected refugees and their non-exposed children: a review of risk and protective factors for trauma transmission. *Psychiatry Research*, *313*, 114604. https://doi.org/10.1016/j.psychres.2022.114604

Kiwan, D. (2019). Inclusion and citizenship: Syrian and Palestinian refugees in Lebanon. *International Journal of Inclusive Education*, *25*(2), 1–15. https://doi.org/10.1080/13603116.2019.1707308

Manduchi, P. (2021). Lebanon, confessionalism, protests: challenging the ancient regime. [online] *esteri.it*. Italy: UNIMED – Unione delle Università del Mediterraneo. Available at: https://www.esteri.it/wp-content/uploads/2021/12/Unimed_Per-unanalisi-delle-proteste-libanesi.pdf (accessed March 3, 2023).

Morina, N., Schnyder, U., Klaghofer, R., Müller, J. and Martin-Soelch, C. (2018). Trauma exposure and the mediating role of post-traumatic stress on somatic symptoms in civilian war victims. *BMC Psychiatry*, *18*(1). doi:https://doi.org/10.1186/s12888-018-1680-4

Naal, H., Nabulsi, D., El Arnaout, N., Abdouni, L., Dimassi, H., Harb, R. and Saleh, S. (2021). Prevalence of depression symptoms and associated sociodemographic and clinical correlates among Syrian refugees in Lebanon. *BMC Public Health*, *21*(1). https://doi.org/10.1186/s12889-021-10266-1

Norris, A.E. and Aroian, K.J. (2008). Avoidance symptoms and assessment of posttraumatic stress disorder in Arab immigrant women. *Journal of Traumatic Stress*, [online] *21*(5), 471–478. doi:https://doi.org/10.1002/jts.20363

Norris, J., Sawyer, R.D. and Lund, D. (2012). *Duoethnography*. New York: Oxford University Press.

OHCHR (2021). *Experts of the Committee on the Elimination of Racial Discrimination Ask Lebanon about the Kafala System for Migrant Domestic Workers, the Absence of a Definition of Racial Discrimination, and the Treatment of Refugees*. [online] OHCHR. Available at: https://www.ohchr.org/en/press-releases/2021/08/experts-committee-elimination-racial-discrimination-ask-lebanon-about-kafala (accessed May 23, 2023).

Popham, C.M., McEwen, F.S., Karam, E., Fayyad, J., Karam, G., Saab, D., Moghames, P. and Pluess, M. (2022). The dynamic nature of refugee children's resilience: a cohort study of Syrian refugees in Lebanon. *Epidemiology and Psychiatric Sciences*, [online] *31*(e41). https://doi.org/10.1017/s2045796022000191

Puig, N. (2020). The Shatila soundscape: Sound cultures, practices, and perceptions in a refugee camp in Lebanon. *Violence: An International Journal*, *1*(2), 285–302 https://doi.org/10.1177/2633002420961399.

Rusdi, A. (2016). Patience in Islamic psychology and its measurement. In conference paper submission for the 3rd Inter-Islamic University Confrence on Psychology. Universitas Islam Indonesia.

Sack, M., Lahmann, C., Jaeger, B. and Henningsen, P. (2007). Trauma Prevalence and Somatoform Symptoms. *The Journal of Nervous and Mental Disease*, *195*(11), 928–933. https://doi.org/10.1097/nmd.0b013e3181594846
Schnitker, S.A., Houltberg, B., Dyrness, W. and Redmond, N. (2017). The virtue of patience, spirituality, and suffering: integrating lessons from positive psychology, psychology of religion, and Christian theology. *Psychology of Religion and Spirituality*, *9*(3), 264–275. doi:https://doi.org/10.1037/rel0000099.
Schwarz, S. (2018). Resilience in psychology: a critical analysis of the concept. *Theory & Psychology*, *28*(4), 528–541. https://doi.org/10.1177/0959354318783584.
Southwick, S.M., Bonanno, G.A., Masten, A.S., Panter-Brick, C. and Yehuda, R. (2014). Resilience definitions, theory, and challenges: interdisciplinary perspectives. *European Journal of Psychotraumatology*, *5*(1), 25338. https://doi.org/10.3402/ejpt.v5.25338.
Theisen-Womersley, G. (2021). Collective trauma, collective healing. In *Trauma and Resilience Among Displaced Populations*. Cham: Springer, 147–173. https://doi.org/10.1007/978-3-030-67712-1_6.
UNHCR (2022). *UNHCR in Lebanon*. [online] UNHCR.org. Available at: https://www.unhcr.org/countries/lebanon (accessed February 12, 2023).
World Bank (2021). *Population, total – Lebanon | Data*. [online] data.worldbank.org. Available at: https://data.worldbank.org/indicator/SP.POP.TOTL?locations=LB (accessed February 10, 2023).

10

CAPTURE THE MOMENT

Art Therapy Practical Training with Older People who have Dementia

Raquel Chapin Stephenson and Eha Rüütel

Abstract

This study examines the experience of arts therapy student trainees in practical training with older people who have dementia. The study was a component of the Arts Therapies Dementia Project of Estonia, which trained new creative arts therapists with the skills needed to work with older adults with dementia. The principles of critical participatory action research with an emphasis on experiential learning and the process of reflection were followed in the course of the training. Thirteen trainees, women aged 24–60 (eight specialists and five masters students) completed the training. The data was captured after the completion of the traineeship by a semi-structured questionnaire that was developed during the training, which aimed to describe trainees' expectations, professional development and teamwork. Conventional content analysis revealed four categories describing 1) expectations; 2) challenges; 3) therapists' and clients' memories; and 4) trainees' coping and the impact of the traineeship.

The study found that experiential learning was relevant and valuable and supported learners in discovering the nuances of therapeutic presence and developing the necessary key skills to work with older adults with impaired memory. As a result of this study, the student collaborative practice in a nursing home became a part of the arts therapies master's programme of Tallinn University. Future research might explore influences on the formation of the intra-specialty choices and the trajectory of skill development to competent practitioners of arts therapies students.

Keywords: experiential learning, participatory action research, arts therapies, art therapy, older adults, dementia, memory loss

DOI: 10.4324/9781032663944-10

Abstract in Estonian

Käesolevas uuringus käsitletakse kunstiteraapiate eriala praktikantide kogemusi dementsusega eakatega Eestis. See uuring oli osa Eesti projektist, mille käigus koolitati uusi loovterapeute, kellel on oskused töötada dementsusega eakatega. Koolituse käigus järgiti kriitilise osalus-tegevusuuringu põhimõtteid rõhuasetusega kogemuslikul õppimisel ja refleksiooni protsessil. Koolituse läbis 13 praktikanti, naised vanuses 24–60 aastat (8 spetsialisti ja 5 magistranti). Andmed koguti pärast praktika läbimist poolstruktureeritud küsimustikuga, mis töötati välja koolituse käigus ja mille eesmärk oli kirjeldada praktikantide ootusi, professionaalset arengut ja meeskonnatööd. Tavapärane sisuanalüüs tõi välja neli kategooriat, mis kirjeldavad 1) ootusi, 2) väljakutsed, 3) terapeutide ja klientide mälestusi ning 4) praktikantide toimetulekut ja praktika mõju. Uuringus leiti, et kogemuslik õppimine oli asjakohane ja väärtuslik ning toetas õppijaid terapeutilise kohaloleku nüansside avastamisel ja vajalike võtmeoskuste arendamisel halvenenud mäluga vanemaealistega töötamiseks. Selle uuringu tulemusena kujunes üliõpilaste koostöine hooldekodus läbiviidav praktika Tallinna Ülikooli kunstiteraapiate magistriõppe osaks. Edaspidi vajaksid uurimist kunstiteraapiate üliõpilaste erialasiseste valikute mõjutajad ja oskuste arengutee pädeva praktikuni.

Introduction

Dementia, designated as a public health priority by the World Health Organization (2021), impacts 50 million people worldwide and that figure is growing by 10 million new cases per year. There is a dire need for trained professionals to care for those suffering from a disease which robs people of their cognitive and, eventually, their physical functioning. Through the practice and examination of an arts therapies internship experience at a nursing home in Estonia, mutual learning occurred for student interns, participants and nursing home staff. This paper will discuss a participatory action research study that took place with the psychoeducational training programme of arts therapies students at Tallinn University and illuminate potential opportunities for future training in dementia care. The research questions were: 1) what do arts therapies student interns face when working with older people with dementia? and 2) how do arts therapies student interns interpret their experience?

This study was a component of the Arts Therapies Dementia Project of Estonia, which trained new arts therapists with the skills needed to work with older adults with memory loss and dementia. Funded by the Estonian Ministry of Social Affairs and the US Embassy in Estonia, it was the first programme of its kind in the country. The one-year course was offered as an elective for graduate arts therapy students at Tallinn University and masters-level professionals. The practical training gave students the opportunity to experiment with methods, tools and approaches that can be used with clients. Moreover, the reflective process allowed them to learn and reflect upon new information in a personal and meaningful way, broadening the opportunity for critical reflection and deepening the construction of meaning (Chen Tsai, 2013; Grushka, 2005). The training promoted the trainees' capacity for reflection by identifying and processing surprises, mistakes and *a-ha* moments (Deaver and Shiflett, 2011), valuing the students as makers of their own knowledge (McAuliffe and Eriksen, 2011), but was also aimed to rework their prior knowledge (Binson and Lev-Wiesel, 2018).

Dementia care

Memory loss and dementia are complex and often devastating experiences that profoundly impact individuals and their families. The experience of memory loss and dementia encompasses a gradual erosion of memories, skills and independence, leading to a sense of identity loss (D'cruz, 2021). The common focus on loss and disability, however, fuels the belief that these symptoms are what define a person's experience and identity (Dupuis, *et al.*, 2012). Research indicates that despite memory loss, self-continuity remains to some degree (Mentzou, *et al.*, 2023; Strikwerda-Brown, *et al.*, 2019), which has important implications for approaches to caregiving and interacting with a person experiencing memory loss. While there does not yet exist a cure for the underlying cause of some forms of dementia (such as Alzheimer's disease), there are ways to improve the quality of life of affected individuals. It is an accepted opinion that treatment of dementia should aim to enhance quality of life and also improve a sense of personhood, mood and behaviour (World Health Organization, 2017).

The care of older adults with dementia in Estonia has traditionally relied on family caregivers. However, the multidimensional nature of caring for an older family member and the accompanying workload for the family is not commonly acknowledged (Laidmäe, *et al.*, 2012), and problems related to the care of people with dementia and caregivers' needs for support have remained unchanged during the last 10–15 years (Varik, Saks and Medar, 2018). Discussions over the last ten years at the community, municipal, professional and national level have focused on the burden of care, access to services and the need for training of caregivers of people with dementia. Thus, in recent years, there have been improvements in care homes that have been adapted to meet the needs of those with dementia. However, specialised training of healthcare professionals to work with people who have dementia, including arts therapists, has been limited if not non-existent.

Arts therapies

Communication is a basic human need. When a person loses the ability to process language and words become an impossible tool for communication, that person is at greater risk for decreased health and well-being. Research shows that psychosocial treatment of dementia improves cognition, quality of life for patient and family caregivers, and the reduction of neuropsychiatric symptoms (Logsdon and Teri, 2018), helping patients to "becom[e] a person again" (Hunter *et al.*, 2016).

The arts therapies can be especially beneficial to an older person with dementia. This expressive psychosocial approach can improve self-esteem and promote a sense of belonging through embodied communication that fosters meaningful engagement (Kontos and Grigorovich, 2018). One powerful aspect of the arts therapies is that communication occurs in the realm of expression encompassing visual language, music and movement. Giving an alternative means to communicate relieves the burden of language impairment or barriers and reduces stress-related behaviours (Mimica and Dubravka, 2011). Zaidel's (2013) research shows that the communicative nature of art is neuronally more damage-resistant than language, and communication through art can have a lasting, positive impact on mental alertness, increased sociability and improved physical and social engagement. Jeppson *et al.* (2022) demonstrated that participating in painting sessions led to improved self-rating of quality of life and increased levels of engagement and communication. In a systemic review of the literature, Emblad and Mukaetova-Ladinska (2021) found that arts therapies that focused on "in the moment" interventions improved cognitive functions, reduced biological and psychological symptoms of dementia, improved well-being and increased quality of life.

Experiential geriatric training

Experiential learning can change perceptions, improve attitudes and communication and increase the cultural and situational sensitivity of students. Conti *et al.* (2016) found that through experience with older adults, students of medicine, nursing, occupational therapy and pharmacy learnt about and appreciated the roles of other professionals, gained practice skills and developed a positive attitude towards older patients. Kitwood (1997) asserted that training through experiential learning, which includes action, reflection and consolidation, creates reflective practitioners. Students were surprised by how the common stereotypes of ageing were overturned in their observation of these active older adults. It is notable that more than 80% of the participants placed a high value on the active experiential component in their overall education.

While the increased focus on dementia has produced more resources available to arts therapists training to work with older adults in recent years, theoretical resources alone are insufficient. Therefore, experiential learning directly with older adults is the most impactful approach to developing awareness, capacity and competency to work with their unique needs. Those who engage in practical training are more likely to gain an improved attitude and develop a greater interest in working with older adults (Bergman *et al.*, 2014). There is an urgent need for arts therapists who specialise in geriatric care. At a time when societal attitudes about ageing continue to be driven by fear, denial and avoidance of death, geriatric-focused experiential training is the best path to increase the chance that students will choose an age-related career (Hash *et al.*, 2017). Ierardi and Goldberg (2014) analysed a seven-week training programme where graduate-level students of health professions, including arts therapists, worked in interprofessional teams four days per week at a community site and spent one day each week in presentations, workshops and small group discussions. This experience seemed to either reinforce students' interest in working with marginalised populations or led them in that direction through didactic and practical experiences. The authors stress that interprofessional learning opportunities foster the development of clinicians who acknowledge their clients' sociocultural differences and systemic interactions.

Method

Study design

The study followed the principles of critical participatory action research, which is defined as "a social process of collaborative learning for the sake of individual and collective self-formation, realised by groups of people who join together in changing the practices through which they interact in a shared social world" (Kemmis *et al.*, 2014, p. 20). By understanding their practices as the product of particular circumstances, participatory action researchers become alert to clues about how it may be possible to transform the practices they are producing and reproducing through their current ways of working. Focusing on practices in a concrete and specific way makes them accessible for reflection, discussion and reconstruction as products of past circumstances that are capable of being modified in and for present and future circumstances.

Intervention description

The one-year Arts Therapies Dementia Project consisted of four overlapping phases that were repeated according to the personal learning needs of the trainees. Phase One included a training programme for 30 trainees – arts therapists, graduate arts therapy students, psychologists and social workers working with people with dementia in care facilities. The two-week training included lectures and workshops on the general principles of psychological and physical ageing; an introduction to arts therapies; creative ageing, including self-help methods; reminiscence work in therapy and counselling; development of an empathic understanding of the world of people with dementia; and methods of assessment of arts therapies. In phase two, arts therapies programming and experiential practice was implemented at four partner institutions. Two of the partnering institutions were day centres for older adults and two were residential care homes. These partnerships also provided an ongoing internship placement for Tallinn University's graduate arts therapies. Each of the 30 trainees conducted 40 therapy sessions, 45 minutes in duration, of individual or group work with older adults with dementia. Sessions were varied by student and participant group, with media choice ranging from 2D to 3D, and structured and unstructured art-making activities depending on the interests, goals and needs of the participant(s). Data was gathered in phase three, including the questionnaire about students' experiences of working with older adults with dementia which is the focus of this article. Phase four was the dissemination of programme outcomes via publications in local newspapers, a methodological e-book and local and international conferences.

The aim of the data gathering of phase three was to understand the experiences of trainees.

The application of the arts therapies varies significantly between different client groups. Thus, both as an apprentice and as a professional, there is a high probability of meeting clients for whom theoretical knowledge of how to do something does not provide sufficient preparation for real therapy work. In particular, this study reveals the complex situations in therapy practice that may occur for a novice therapist. An open discussion about defining oneself as a therapist and analysing one's own unique experiences, thereby developing one's therapeutic awareness and coping with complex situations, supports the participant in the learning process and can lead to valuable pieces of learning for others working with the same client group.

Participants

The 13 trainees who were included in the study were not employed by the partnering institutions, completed the full didactic and experiential traineeship, and completed the questionnaire. Participants were all women between the ages of 24 and 60 (average age 40.6), 8 of them specialists (average age 45.3) and 5 masters students (average age 33.2). Nine of the participants specialised in art therapy, two in dance movement therapy, and one in music therapy, one of the participants was a physiotherapist and one a counselling psychologist. The latter two had training in the implementation of creative methods in therapy and all of them used other modalities in addition to their main art form of therapy. As the respondents' answers described a general human experience rather than the specific effect of the media used, we decided to include the analysis of the questionnaires of all trainees who met the selection criteria, regardless of creative art specialisation. All participants were "beginning students" in the CAT practice with the older adults with dementia because they had not worked with this target group and had previously been exposed to dementia in the elderly either within the family (2) or in connection with a job (1) or previous studies (1).

Measurements

The data was captured by a semi-structured questionnaire that was developed during the training course and based on the feedback of the students and the topics brought to supervision. The topics of the questionnaire were chosen in a discussion with trainees and related open-ended questions were based on the trainees' interests and practice experience. The analysis of self-experience included the following sections: expectations related to the target group (e.g., thoughts, feelings and expectations with which they started working with clients), professional development (e.g., complex situations, perceived failures, emotions and associations noticed during practice; coping with them and assistance received; personal resources discovered in the work with the client group; the most important learning experience).

The questionnaire was emailed to the trainees after the completion of the traineeship. The trainees were interested in completing the questionnaire in order to gain additional perspective of their own experience and that of others.

Ethical considerations

All trainees participated in the study voluntarily and gave their informed consent to use their replies for the purposes of this study. Each participant was assigned a pseudonym. The questionnaire was developed in cooperation with the participants of the study, and the selected topics were important to the participants themselves and in learning about the experiences of others. The focus of the questionnaire lies in the experience of the trainees and did not include the personal data of arts therapy clients.

The participation of the clients was voluntary, and extra care was given to ensure their understanding of the project and any expectations. The institutions participating in the study gave their permission for the study and were informed of the trainees being questioned in order to collect data. Ongoing verbal consent from therapy participants was obtained as part of the invitation process with each session. An overview of the results was introduced to the trainees and participating institutions at the final seminar of the project. The Arts Therapies Dementia Project was supported by Tallinn University and the Estonian Ministry of Social Affairs.

Data analysis

The interview transcripts yielded rich descriptions of trainee experiences. Trainees offered an honest and, at times, vulnerable account of the challenges they encountered. The qualitative analysis was carried out as a conventional content analysis, following the topics of the questionnaire generated in the discussions with students. Conventional content analysis is suitable for the study design, which aims to describe a phenomenon (Hsieh and Shannon, 2005), in the current study the experiences of trainees meeting a new client group. As the questions were answered in some cases more broadly, highlighting information that complemented the answers to other questions, the questionnaire was first read to gain a feel of the essence of the participants' description of their experience. The coded text was then grouped by the questionnaire topics forming the main categories and initial coding scheme. Under each category, the codes were sorted into sub-categories. The sub-categories were illustrated with quotations from the respondents. Minor linguistic corrections were made to the quotations used to illustrate the sub-categories, preserving the characteristic style of presentation of the respondent. Subsequently, the analysis was shared with trainees to ensure accuracy.

Results

Below is a description of the data according to the four categories of inquiry: 1) expectations, 2) challenges, 3) therapists' and clients' memories, and 4) trainees' coping and the impact of the traineeship.

Category one: expectations

We explored how the trainees' expectations changed. The expectations of six of the respondents were related to the ability to test in real life what they had learnt during the training course, curiosity and a wish to positively influence the condition of the client. Seven participants noted that they were emotionally unsure about themselves and the client group before the traineeship. However, their expectations changed throughout the traineeship, becoming more confident and positive about working with older adults. Anu explained her feelings, "I started with anticipation [and] anxiety over a new situation, sensing my responsibility and not knowing my capabilities and abilities to react in unexpected situations . . . [then] the first meetings gave me knowledge that making contact, involvement, understanding and sensing very different worlds is not as hard as I thought."

Similarly, before the first session, Raili said, "I had conflicting feelings. Fear and uncertainty were high. The stories I had heard of various care homes had made me very anxious. I was expecting something quite terrible." However, her feelings quickly changed after the first session, "I felt as if I had received a huge and awaited gift. I can't describe how much joy I felt after the session."

All the trainees questioned, regardless of their expectations, described their first therapy session as positive. Only Elena described also fear of failure and, although she discovered a resource to handle the therapy session during her practice, she was also the only one who indicated that she did not wish to continue working with older adults.

Category two: challenges

Based on the responses provided, challenges had three sub-categories: difficult situations, failures and role confusion.

The trainees stated that there were more *difficult situations* at the beginning because they lacked confidence in their abilities, and the clients had to be persuaded to participate. Trainees learnt that they needed to carry out therapeutic activities considering the needs of the client, such as slow pace and rest. For instance, Maarja described her excessive eagerness to involve a client, "I completely wore out the client, didn't give them time to adjust. We worked for too long and too intensively." Mari describes her awkwardness when the client's thoughts changed in the middle of the sentence or the client lost contact with the therapy situation and started packing oil pastels into paper one by one to hide them.

Difficult moments also included: times when it seemed that there would never be a change in the client's process; when there was doubt regarding the extent to which a therapist can guide or get involved in the work of a client; understanding a client who was unable to express themselves verbally; and normalising situations in which the clients claimed incompetence or saw their work as too primitive. Group work posed a unique difficulty, with several clients needing to be guided/helped at the same time.

In general, what the trainees saw as failures were situations where they felt they did not manage the situation and were related to the therapist's working style and means and methods. The situations students determined as unsuccessful can be also named as important learning experiences, as trainees emphasised the benefit for professional development in the questionnaire.

Learning experience in working style included: a working pace that was too fast, causing confusion and anxiety in the clients; activities of therapists working together that conflicted with each other; involving too many people in group work; starting a therapy session with insufficient preparation and background information; and helping a client too much in activities. For instance, Katrin describes her experience: "Art-related activities were often unpleasant for the client (they were convinced they had no talent and could not handle it) and when I proposed to start drawing or painting straight away, the client got scared and became anxious. Each session should first be started with an introductory conversation . . . finding out how they are feeling today, etc." Kristina noted, "One time we were making a collage and I tried to quicken the work of one of the older adults by helping them colour the background with a pencil. The client was so hurt . . . I learned that what seems right to me, may not be right for the client. I have to let them move at their own pace, even slowly, at their speed. The therapy is meant for them, not for me."

Learning experiences due to the choice of means and methods can be divided into sub-categories: exercises and tasks, materials and display of artwork. The trainees identified the need to give simple and clear tasks. For instance, Raili noted, "The trickiest part was to find a simple way to guide the exercises. Giving options confused the clients." Likewise, Maarja reflected, "Tasks related to emotions and self-perception failed completely." Failures arose from providing materials that were too hard to handle. For instance, Anu described, "Small sticky images consisting of tiny pieces that were difficult to pick up and see." Kadri also noted, "It was also difficult to work with materials that seemed edible. In activities with modelling paste, there was a possibility it might be eaten." In displaying artwork, a safe place for exhibition had to be found. Liis wrote, "We placed the client's works on the wall above their bed and their roommate ripped them off at one point. That taught us that it is not a good idea to place the work in a client's room in a care home if they share the room. It is better to have an exhibition." Inevitability also had a role to play in the important experiences. Heli noted: "Due to personal plans, I had to take a break from working with the clients. In the meantime, one of them passed away and we could never do some of the activities we had planned."

Category three: therapists' and clients' memories

Trainees' personal memories led to unexpected situations of role confusion. The role confusion could be divided into three sub-categories: confusion in therapist-client relationship related to generations; unexpected feelings; and confusing associations related to oneself and loved ones.

Generational confusion between a client and a practitioner was described in both directions. Heli noted, "There were moments when some people started reminding me of someone close to me from the older generation." Triin recalled,

"Sometimes, the older adults acted as if I was a child. That, in turn, made me want to be a good child and to avoid uncomfortable topics."

Regarding unexpected feelings, the respondents described how they took over the feelings of the clients. Anu wrote of "[. . .] sadness about the client who always wept when I left, who wanted a lot of physical contact that, at the same time, made the client cry even more." Elena reflected, "On several occasions, I sensed how terrible it would be to relive the painful memories over and over again." And, Kristina described her arising feelings, "I became slow myself, got tired quickly, felt old." There were fewer instances of positive emotions and these were mostly related to successful artworks of clients or to general attitudes towards older people. Elena stated, "I experienced joy and lightness when the artwork brought positive emotions to the clients and made them happy – they lightened up, laughed, enjoyed creating and communicating and made jokes." Raili remarked, "Since I like elderly people very much, I felt warmth, wisdom and kindness when working with them."

Trainees' associations with themselves or loved ones were related to: a) hindsight – Mari wrote, "I often thought of my father who is already dead;" b) existential thoughts about life, death or loneliness; c) fears regarding the future of oneself and loved ones getting old, being lonely or seeing one's parents getting old; d) guilt about placing a loved one in a care home – Maarja noted, "I was probably trying to ease my guilt with this traineeship, to transfer what I failed to do for my loved one;" and e) gratefulness, as described by Mari, "I feel grateful that my elderly mother can be on her own at home."

Category four: trainees' coping and the impact of the traineeship

In addition to supportive supervision and cooperation with the care team, the trainees acknowledged working a great deal on themselves during the traineeship. Difficult situations were easier to handle by becoming more self-aware and acknowledging role confusion. Prior experience, skills gained during the traineeship, and professional literature also helped. Students felt that coping highlighted personal resources such as patience, calmness, authenticity, simplicity, empathy, ability to listen, sensitivity, kindness, humour, friendliness, personal communication skills, clear voice and expression, positive attitude, resourcefulness, courage, attentiveness, adaptation to the client's reality and acceptance. Trainees mentioned that certain strategic activities were used for self-regulation during the sessions: viewing the situation from the side, staying calm, focusing on one thing at a time, turning the focus of a client from negative to positive, moving step by step, communicating on an adult-to-adult level. There were simple things that helped to cope with difficulties.

According to Heli, "It was useful to know who should sit next to who, the background information of the people, who needs special assistance, etc." And, Elena noted, "After the sessions, restorative actions were used: sharing emotions, reflection with the co-therapist, writing, dancing and other creative activities."

Despite difficult situations, all of the respondents considered the traineeship a valuable experience, even when the trainee did not wish to work with this population in the future.

Complexity of memory and identity

When getting to know the particularities of older adults with dementia, the trainees discovered that the phenomenon of memory loss is not a complete and one-way process, as noted by Raili: "although they may have forgotten why they came here in the middle of the dance movement session, they were extremely precise and skillful in reflecting movements. For me, it was proof that they still have body memory. By stimulating body memory, making contacts can be made easier and communication may take place via movement, thus decreasing the impact of verbal and cognitive difficulties." Links between memory and identity were discovered, for example. Triin noted, "Identity is usually linked to memory . . . when the memory has been (partially) lost and knowledge about oneself have thus become inaccessible, art can be used to communicate. By reflecting this back, the therapist can help the person become aware of themselves." Maarja wrote, "I learnt to acknowledge the unique identity of older adults with dementia."

Staying in the present

The trainees gained experience in, "maintaining contact by using the present moment, noticing wishes and needs, discomfort, stress and anxiety-inducing situations and how these are expressed in their body language, attitudes and emotions," as explained by Elena. "There was a need to be spontaneously creative, flexible, calm and ready for surprises," according to Heli. The trainees learnt how to be clear in their intentions and descriptions regarding art materials and the structure of a session. It was collaborative learning by doing, as described by Raili, "The (older women) in the group taught me how to explain things in a simpler and calmer way."

Cooperation with older adults with dementia required critical self-observation and a willingness to change, as described by Elena, "It is important to monitor the pace . . . At first, it was very difficult to assess how much slower and calmer I needed to be. It seemed to me that I was calm and speaking slowly and simply, but the pace was still too high for the client. It took several sessions to start sensing and understanding this group." Maarja reflected, "Little by little, I got the skill of being patient, slow, learned to stop myself from doing all the work for the clients, gave them a possibility to decide for themselves."

The traineeship also had a larger impact. Anna, who had prior experience in taking care of a family member with dementia admitted after the traineeship, "I believe that I could connect with the family member better now." Eliisa emphasised the importance of a learning experience in an institution, "I learnt how employees used communication to cope with their highly stressful work."

Discussion

The experiential training provided a rich learning opportunity and illuminated several key aspects of the unique qualities and challenges that arise for emerging practitioners in their work with older people with dementia. Similar to the research by Conti *et al.* (2016) and Bergman *et al.* (2014), the trainees' reflections on their experiential learning highlighted an improved attitude and a greater interest in working with older adults. Working in the institutions gave trainees the opportunity to learn about the roles of other professionals and experience the interprofessional collaboration stressed also by Conti *et al.* (2016) and Ierardi and Goldberg (2014).

The survey conducted at the end of the training gave trainees the opportunity to reflect on the practical experience gained during the course and to combine it with theoretical knowledge. Their responses highlighted the specific value of experiential learning, that knowledge is consolidated through practical experience, and that all "self-evident" (small) things need to be tested in a therapeutic context. The reflective process allowed them to digest the information in a more personal and meaningful way and gave opportunity for critical reflection as previous studies (Chen Tsai, 2013; Deaver and Shiflett, 2011; Grushka, 2005; and Schmid and Rolvsjord, 2021) have shown. Experiential learning helps to fill the gap between theory and practice in academic learning and creates an opportunity for new knowledge to emerge (Binson and Lev-Wiesel, 2018).

The aim of the study was to identify the critical topics of art therapy students' internships. We approached this with two research questions: 1) what do arts therapy student interns face when working with older people with dementia? 2) how do arts therapy student interns interpret their experience? An analysis of the data revealed two main themes: firstly, the need to develop key skills needed to work with older adults, and secondly, discovering therapeutic presence alongside memory loss. These themes will be discussed below.

The core of the reflections seems to be the therapeutic presence (Geller and Greenberg, 2012), and the ability to capture the moment. Colosimo and Pos (2015) present a rational model of the therapeutic presence, which includes "being here," "being now," "being open" and "being with-and-for the client".

Schwarz *et al.* (2018) identified the following component themes of therapeutic presence in art therapy: attentive focus, joining, movement, uncertainty and sense of completeness. The art therapists interviewed emphasised the importance of preparation for the session and the role of art in all main areas of the art therapist's therapeutic presence. Tannen *et al.* (2019), according to the results of their study with counsellors in training, describe a model of continuum – a continuous, moment-to-moment process, where trainees either seek safety by acting to contain their anxiety and uncertainty or seek connection by choosing to be more present. The choices take place in contexts that either inhibit or facilitate being present, including trainees' knowledge, skills and experiences.

Theme one: development of skills

The growth of the trainees was apparent as they learned through experience to adapt their communication and pacing to the older adult and dealt with difficulties. Though they often saw the outcome of their work as a failure, it was also an important learning moment, where deep self-awareness occurred, "seeing" the elderly in more focus and gaining confidence to move through a difficult moment and find success. Thus, promoting the capacity for self-reflection and shaping/making their own knowledge, as also noted by McAuliffe and Eriksen (2011) and Schmid and Rolvsjord (2021). Trainees learnt the importance of attunement (Kossak, 2021), to be present and alert to the moment. Trainees' personal memories and associations related to older people and their condition sometimes diverted attention and interrupted the therapeutic presence. However, step by step, trainees became more aware of factors influencing the quality of the therapy session. They learnt to understand the client's non-verbal and emotional reactions, for example, by paying close attention to how the participant moves a paintbrush across the paper or slowly and carefully presses their fingers into a ball of clay. With increasing experience, trainees learnt how to create the right amount of structure in the arts therapies session to engage and retain the attention of the clients, altering their pacing, which included speaking and moving more slowly and allowing more time for clients to respond. Trainees learnt how to adapt art-making to encourage the client's freedom of expression within a safe, organised, successful structure. By carefully planning the art-making tools and activity to be purposefully scaffolded, participants could experience art-making within the realm of their cognitive and physical functionality. In this way, the trainees' work with their older clients fostered a supportive psychosocial experience that enhanced communication and promoted authentic expression (Stephenson, 2021). Valuing the individual as a whole person, not seeing them only as a diagnosis of dementia and operating in a way that promotes meaningful engagement and a life worth living are essential components of person-centred care for those with dementia (Stephenson, 2021).

Theme two: discovering therapeutic presence alongside memory loss

Role confusion emerged during the training, highlighting the ongoing importance of confronting biases and beliefs about ourselves and others. At times negative associations of ageing emerged, and students were faced with confronting their attitudes and, at times, their actions. Though difficult to address, this second theme illuminated how vital confronting ageism is in gerontology training (Friedman and Goldbaum, 2016). Key to the students' development was learning how to see the identity of their client despite the symptoms of memory loss, such as observing body memory or recognising the link between memory and sense of self. Students created new possibilities to support, care for and relate to people with memory loss, counteracting the "tragedy discourse" of doom and disability (Dupuis, *et al.*, 2016). Students became more aware of and confronted confusion regarding their role as arts therapists. Throughout the traineeship, they deepened their engagement with the clients and it became easier to maintain a therapeutic presence – being here, now, open and in communion (Colosimo and Pos, 2015). In line with the findings of Schwarz *et al.* (2018), over the course of several months working with the clients, trainees became more intuitive, softer and authentic and trusting their ability to attune to their clients.

Another common theme was the hesitation to work with older adults at the outset of the training, with mixed feelings about older adults. However, after getting to know the clients, building their own skills and expanding their capacity for self-reflection and growth through experiential learning (Kitwood, 1997; Deaver and Shiflett, 2011), the trainees' attitudes improved (Bergman, *et al.*, 2014). The contrast of the before/after expectations/experiences of the trainees speaks to the power of experiential learning to challenge a person's preconceived notions in ways that the textbook, lecture and discussion do not.

Impact on curriculum and implementation

An important result of this action research was the recognition that with the older target group arts therapy students definitely need practical experience during their studies. Owing to the ageing society, art therapy carried out in nursing homes with the target group of older adults will definitely be an important field of work in the future. That's why Tallinn University's arts therapies masters studies include an internship in a nursing home, which is completed in the middle of the two-year study when the initial internship experiences have already been acquired. This practice requires specific preparation both in terms of the cognitive and physical health of older people, as well as the readiness for the therapy process to be interrupted due to the health problems or death of the elder client. Since the survey revealed that it was necessary to deal with what happened in the session immediately, the internship at the nursing home is structured as a collaborative one, where at least two arts therapies students (preferably from art therapy and dance movement therapy, allowing the integration of different modalities) are in the internship at the same time. This encourages thinking and planning therapy sessions together and enables reflection and mutual analysis of experiences immediately after the session.

To ensure the success of the cooperation process, we have chosen a nursing home as the internship base, where students can also live during the internship. This approach of intensive cooperation is similar to that described by Ierardi and Goldberg (2014), where they pointed out that collaborative practical experience with a certain target group reinforced interest in working with that target group. The internship experience so far allows us to conclude that it also supports the study group as a whole, generating common memories and coping experiences. The two-week presence in the nursing home expands the possibilities for planning the time of therapy sessions based on the mood and wishes of the clients and the daily schedule of the institution. It also allows for more and longer sessions in nature, as the nursing home is located in a naturally beautiful location.

It is very important to leave time in the session for a conversation if the client needs it. Arts therapies bring to mind familiar activities from the past (artwork, crafts, natural materials, singing, listening to music and moving in music) and related stories, the important task of the therapist is to take time for listening (Stephenson, 2021). By going at the same pace of life as the residents of the nursing home, it is easier to acquire a slow pace, simple and clear self-expression and other important aspects of working with the elderly, regarding activities and art materials. Being in the same environment also facilitates a therapeutic presence, and trainees find it easier to manage their memories and parallels with everyday life and loved ones.

Limitations of the study

The Arts Therapies Dementia Project demonstrated the multifaceted benefits of co-creating knowledge through experiential learning. However, there are several limitations to this study. While trainees gave thoughtful feedback on their experiences on a range of topics, the sample size is small and includes the viewpoints only of women. We received anecdotal feedback from clients and their families, however, a more formal assessment of the client experience was not conducted. While the trainee perspective is valuable to establish a deeper understanding of the participatory educational experience, knowing about the client experience would be a valuable contribution to the overall evaluation of the impact of the trainees' work. Additional biases are likely to exist, as the trainees' understanding of their clients are seen from their own personal, cultural and generational lens. Additionally, we did not ask about the topics that older adults with dementia brought to the arts therapies sessions. Thus, this research, which was focused on the trainees' experiences, does not provide insight into the issues of older adults with dementia that arose during therapy.

Implications for practice

Further research could focus more closely on arts therapists who are working in the field to find out how the choice of specialty took place and to better understand the trajectory from skill development to competent practitioner. This would provide an opportunity to better guide and support students' choices for arts therapies for the elderly and elderly with dementia during their studies. Although there has been a rise in the number of arts therapists working in rehabilitation and social care – where elderly people with dementia are one of the target groups – since the project discussed in this article, there is still a need for more focused attention on the needs of those with dementia and how to care for them.

Conclusion

The data gathered from the Dementia Project illuminates how this project trained arts therapies students by improving their skills working with older adults with dementia. Students developed, through critical reflection, the skills to work with the unique pace of the older adult with dementia – to move slowly, pause and give time to adjust in each step. They also learnt how to be present in the moment with each person, not ahead or behind, by carefully monitoring responses, noticing opportunities for cooperation and being curious and supportive. Lastly, the findings of this study are being used to guide the training of arts therapies students.

This study contributes to a growing body of research in the arts therapies that explores how arts therapists learn by doing, while also demonstrating that recognising and addressing bias is vital to the student's development of therapeutic skills. Memory loss is frightening not only to those it directly afflicts but the fear of dementia has a societal impact that has led to stigmatisation (Low and Purwaningrum, 2020). However, as discovered in this study, coming to terms with this stigma must be addressed in the process of developing therapeutic skills. Dementia has been recognised as a top global health concern (WHO, 2021) and it is imperative to educate skilled professionals to tackle this challenge effectively.

References

Bergman, E., Erikson, M.A., and Simons, J. (2014). Attracting and training tomorrow's gerontologists: What drives student interest in aging? *Educational Gerontology, 40*, 172–185. https://doi.org/10.1080/03601277.2013.802184

Binson, B. and Lev-Wiesel, R. (2018). Promoting personal growth through experiential learning: The case of expressive arts therapy for lecturers in Thailand. *Frontiers in Psychology*, *8*. https://doi-org.ezproxyles.flo.org/10.3389/fpsyg.2017.02276

Chen Tsai, K. (2013). Two channels of learning: Transformative learning and creative learning. *American International Journal of Contemporary Research*, 3, 32–37. http://www.aijcrnet.com/journals/Vol_3_No_1_January_2013/5.pdf

Colosimo, K.A. and Pos, A.E. (2015). A rational model of expressed therapeutic presence. *Journal of Psychotherapy Integration*, *25*(2), 100–114. http://dx.doi.org/10.1037/a0038879

Conti, G., Bowers, B., O'Connell, M.B., Bruerd, S., Bugdalski-Strutrud, C., Smith, G., Bickese, J., and Mendes, J. (2016). Examining the effects of an experiential interprofessional education activity with older adults. *Journal of Interprofessional Care*, *30*(2), 184–190. https://doi.org/10.3109/13561820.2015.1092428

D'cruz, M.M. (2021). Does Alice live here anymore? Autonomy and identity in persons living and dying with dementia. *Frontiers in Psychiatry*, *12*. https://doi.org/10.3389/fpsyt.2021.700567

Deaver, S.P. and Shiflett, C. (2011). Art-based supervision techniques. *The Clinical Supervisor*, *30*, 257–276. https://doi.org/10.1080/07325223.2011.619456

Dupuis, S.L., Wiersma, E., and Loiselle, L. (2012). Pathologizing behavior: Meanings of behaviors in dementia. *Journal of Aging Studies, 26*(2), 162–73. https://doi.org/10.1016/j.jaging.2011.12.001

Dupuis, S.L., Kontos, P., Mitchell, G., Jonas-Simpson, C., and Gray, J. (2016). Reclaiming citizenship through the arts. *Dementia*, *15*(3), 358–80. https://doi.org/10.1177/1471301216637206

Emblad, S. and Mukaetova-Ladinska, E. (2021). Creative art therapy as a non-pharmacological intervention for dementia: A systematic review. *Journal of Alzheimer's Disease Reports*, *5*(1), 353–364. https://doi.org/10.3233/adr-201002

Friedman, F.B. and Goldbaum, C.S. (2016). Experiential learning: Developing insights about working with older adults. *Journal of Clinical Social Work*, *44*, 186–197. https://doi.org/10.1007/s10615-016-0583-4

Geller, S.M. and Greenberg, L.S. (2012). *Therapeutic Presence: A Mindful Approach to Effective Therapy.* Washington, DC: American Psychological Association. https://doi.org/10.1037/13485-000

Grushka, K. (2005). Artists as reflective self-learners and cultural communicators: An exploration of the qualitative aesthetic dimension of knowing self through reflective practice in art-making. *Reflective Practice*, *6*, 353–366. https://doi.org/10.1080/14623940500220111

Hash, K.M., Poole, P., Floyd, M., Moore, C.D., Rogers, A.T., and Tower, L.E. (2017). Innovative experiential learning activities in aging: The experiences of four BEL projects. *Journal of Teaching in Social Work*, *37*(2), 156–170. http://dx.doi.org/10.1080/08841233.2017.1300207

Hsieh, H.-F. and Shannon, S.E. (2005). Three approaches to qualitative content analysis. *Qualitative Health Research*, *15*(9), 1277–1288. https://doi.org/10.1177/1049732305276687

Hunter, A., Keady, J., Casey, D., Grealish, A., and Murphy, K. (2016). Psychosocial intervention use in long-stay dementia care: A classic grounded theory. *Qualitative Health Research*, *26*(14), 2024–2034. https://doi:org.ezproxyles.flo.org/10.1177/1049732316632194

Ierardi, F. and Goldberg, E. (2014). Looking back, looking forward: New masters-level creative arts therapists reflect on the professional impact of an interprofessional community health internship. *The Arts in Psychotherapy*, *41*, 366–374. http://dx.doi.org/10.1016/j.aip.2014.06.002

Jeppson, T.A., Nudo, C.A., and Mayer, J.F. (2022). Painting for a purpose: A visual arts program as a method to promote engagement, communication, cognition, and quality of life for individuals with dementia. *American Journal of Speech-Language Pathology, 31*, 1687–1701. https://doi.org/10.1044/2022_AJSLP-21-00300

Kemmis, S., McTaggart, R., and Nixon, R. (2014). *Action Research Planner: Doing Critical Participatory Action Research*. New York, NY: Springer.

Kitwood, T. (1997). *Dementia Reconsidered: The Person Comes First*. Maidenhead: Open University Press. https://doi.org/10.1136/bmj.318.7187.880a

Kontos, P., and Grigorovich, A. (2018). Rethinking musicality in dementia as embodied and relational. *Journal of Aging Studies, 45*, 39–48. https://doi.org/10.1016/j.jaging.2018.01.006

Kossak, M. (2021). *Attunement in Expressive Arts Therapy: Toward an Understanding of Embodied Empathy*. Springfield, IL: Charles C. Thomas.

Laidmäe, V., Tammsaar, K., Tulva, T., and Kasepalu, A. (2012). Quality of life of elderly in Estonia. *The Internet Journal of Geriatrics and Gerontology, 7*(1). https://ispub.com/IJGG/7/1/14023

Logsdon, R.G. and Teri, L. (2018). Quality of life in dementia: Conceptualization, measurement, and psychosocial treatment implications. In G.E. Smith and S.T. Farias (eds.), *APA Handbook of Dementia*, 237–248. Washington, DC: American Psychological Association. https://doi.org/10.1037/0000076-012

Low, L.F. and Purwaningrum, F. (2020). Negative stereotypes, fear and social distance: A systematic review of depictions of dementia in popular culture in the context of stigma. *BMC Geriatrics, 20*, 477. https://doi.org/10.1186/s12877-020-01754-x

McAuliffe, G. and Eriksen, K. (eds.). (2011). *Handbook of Counselor Preparation: Constructivist, Developmental, and Experiential Approaches*. Thousand Oaks, CA: Sage.

Mentzou, A., Sixsmith, J., Ellis, M.P., and Ross, J. (2023). Change in the psychological self in people living with dementia: A scoping review. *Clinical Psychology Review, 101*. https://doi.org/10.1016/j.cpr.2023.102268

Mimica, N. and Dubravka, K. (2011). Art therapy may be beneficial for reducing stress-related behaviours in people with dementia – case report. *Psychiatria Danubina, 23*(1), 125–128.

Schmid, W. and Rolvsjord, R. (2021). Becoming a reflexive practitioner: Exploring music therapy students' learning experiences with participatory role-play in a Norwegian context. *Scandinavian Journal of Educational Research, 65*(5), 864–876. https://doi.org/10.1080/00313831.2020.1755723

Schwarz, N., Snir, S., and Regev, D. (2018). The therapeutic presence of the art therapist. *Art Therapy: Journal of the American Art Therapy Association, 35*(1), 11–18. https://doi.org/10.1080/07421656.2018.1459115

Stephenson, R.C. (2021). *Art Therapy and Creative Aging: Reclaiming Elderhood, Health and Wellbeing*. New York, NY: Routledge.

Strikwerda-Brown, C., Grilli, M., Andrews-Hanna, J., and Irish, M. (2019). "All is not lost"—Rethinking the nature of memory and the self in dementia. *Ageing Research Reviews, 54*. https://doi.org/10.1016/j.arr.2019.100932

Tannen, T., Daniels, M.H., and Koro-Ljungberg, M. (2019). Choosing to be present with clients: an evidence-based model for building trainees' counselling competence. *British Journal of Guidance and Counselling, 47*(4), 405–419. https://doi.org/10.1080/03069885.2017.1370694

Varik, M., Saks, K., and Medar, M. (2018). Dementsusega inimeste ja omastehooldajate vajadused. [The needs of the people with dementia and their caregivers]. *Sotsiaaltöö, 1*, 30–39. Available at: https://www.terviseinfo.ee/et/blogi/5020-dementsusega-inimeste-ja-omastehooldajate-vajadused

World Health Organization (2017). *Global Action Plan on the Public Health Response to Dementia, 2017–2025*. Available at: https://www.who.int/publications/i/item/global-action-plan-on-the-public-health-response-to-dementia-2017---2025 (accessed January 5, 2020).

World Health Organization. (2021). Dementia fact sheet. https://www.who.int/news-room/fact-sheets/detail/dementia (accessed May 4, 2023).

Zaidel, D.W. (2013). Biological and neuronal underpinnings of creativity in the arts. In O. Vartanian, A.S. Bristol and J.C. Kaufman (eds.), *Neuroscience of Creativity*. Cambridge, MA: MIT Press.

11

REFLECTIONS ON IMPLICIT AND EXPLICIT MEMORY IN DRAMA AND MOVEMENT THERAPY

Interview with Aleka Loutsis, Royal Central School of Speech and Drama, University of London, UK

Abstract

This chapter is a transcript of an interview with Aleka Loutsis in October 2023, who reflects on the subject of memory in her work as a dance movement psychotherapist, dramatherapist and teacher. She draws on her substantial experience and elaborates on questions of implicit and explicit memory, cultural expression and reflections on ritual and motif in clinical practice. Loutsis explains how the arts therapies access, shape, and express affective memory and how the body can hold memory before it has reached consciousness. She develops thinking about the developmental gestures (1993) of *yield*, *push*, *reach*, *grasp* and *pull* first outlined by Bainbridge-Cohen as a mapping and language for accessing memories and extending movement repertoire. This is a personal and spontaneous interview, which captures ideas from a pioneer in the field of dance movement therapy and dramatherapy. What emerges through the conversation is a unique approach to working which is intuitive, artistic and relational and above all, processual.

Keywords: implicit memory, explicit memory, developmental gestures, cultural memory, spontaneous movement

Richard Hougham: Thank you for joining me to talk about memory and your work as a dramatherapist and dance movement psychotherapist. The first question I'd like to ask grapples with memory in different ways in terms of the disciplines of the arts therapies and memory as history, testimony, legacy, memory as forgotten. There were so many different strands to the ECArTE conference, which explored this theme, but one of the things that your work has engaged

DOI: 10.4324/9781032663944-11

with over the years is memory in the body. Maybe we can start with that question of how you understand memory and how it relates to the body and movement of the body.

Aleka Loutsis: I realise there are so many ways that you can come to that question. For example, if we consider neuroscientific research in the field of trauma, there is an understanding of how stress is held in the body. This examines muscular tensions and how the nervous system is affected by stress, as well as how it expresses that information through the body, such as in the fight/flight response. This discovery is important to hold in mind as it informs our practice as clinicians. It supports our ongoing assessment and formulation of approach to the therapy. It gives a perspective of what happens in the body, and when I say the body, I am referring to the whole psychobiological system. So, from the extensive research in the field of trauma, there is no question that memory is held in the body. Bessel van der Kolk evidences that clearly in his book *The Body Keeps the Score* (2014) and others have demonstrated how pre-verbal developmental experiences are unconsciously encoded into the system such as in the work of Sue Gerhardt in *Why Love Matters* (2004).

I would like to focus on two types of memory: implicit memory and explicit memory. Implicit memory relates to non-verbal aspects of experience, what you've learnt unconsciously – it's not really in your conscious periphery. Explicit memory on the other hand is conscious. It might be a particular event that you can cognitively remember and call back in. I think the following descriptions found in Ogden, Minton and Pain (2006, p. 236) are helpful: "Implicit memories are best thought of as somatic and affective memory states that are not accompanied by an internal sense that something from the past is being remembered." Whereas, when retrieving explicit memory, "we recall a past experience with a subjective sense that we are remembering something" (op.cit).

You can work with memory from both perspectives. One would be the body holding that which is unknown, perhaps there is a felt sense of something and the movement enables that something to emerge, which may then become more conscious. You might be moving in the presence of a witness, emphasising the relational aspect, providing an opportunity for reflections and potential meaning-making of that embodied movement experience. Or, you can have a particular memory or event that you want to explore, or a dream for example. Dreams may also call in memories. To me what is interesting is how movement can unlock memory stored in the body. Joan Chodorow (1991) describes the significant link between memory and the moving body, "as if certain memories are stored kinaesthetically and can be best retrieved through the movements of the body" (p. 115). She goes on to say that it is our "embodied link to the past" (op. cit.). Our implicit memory is formed pre-verbally, up to 18 months, and is associated with the right hemisphere of the brain, so it concerns body sensations and emotional states. I can talk about that later because it also relates to the developmental gestures and early patterns of behaviour that we learn and how these continue in later life. Explicit memory develops later, around 18–24 months, in a part of the brain that gradually mediates the integration of implicit experience along with the formation of factual and autobiographical memory (Dunlea, 2019, p. 48).

Richard Hougham: Let's just pause on explicit and implicit memory because that is an interesting distinction. It's a philosophical question about the nature of memory and where it comes from. So, just talk a little bit more about implicit and explicit memory.

Aleka Loutsis: Implicit memory is a deeply held and embodied unconscious phenomena. So, we are not aware of it, it is just there. This could also apply to genetically stored transgenerational memory. For example, behaviour can be transmitted from generation to generation at a cellular level, so you could say this too is an unconscious process, something that we are not aware of. So, when I think of implicit memory in that sense, it's a form of imprint that has been generationally passed on by our ancestors. Scientific research in epigenetics, I believe, will eventually prove this idea of transmission between generations. Implicit memory from a developmental perspective relates to pre-verbal stages, including in-utero, through to about 18 months, where the primary relational experience of the infant and caregiver forms initial patterns of attachment and behaviour responses. This relates directly to the quality of contact such as the sensation of being held, the facial expressions, the tone of voice, that whole social engagement system that Stephen Porges (2011) has researched and articulated in *The Polyvagal Theory*. So, while I have discussed two ways that I understand implicit body memory, in my mind there must inevitably be an overlap. What is interesting here are the traces of these experiences, the shapes, sensations and shadow moves outside of our conscious awareness.

Richard Hougham: That is fascinating. It is interesting to think about implicit memory as this potentially cellular inheritance, a genetic transmission or some sort of biological transmission in the body from generation to generation. It brings in questions of inheritance as well, in terms of trauma, in terms of memory of generations. It reminds me, in Yorùbá culture – there is double memory. There is the memory of your life as it's happened and happening and the memories you can recall, which I think would probably be similar to explicit memory, but then there is the second memory, the ancestral memory, which is the memory that you inherit, which is also part of the predisposition of the psyche. It's interesting, these versions of memory which might reach back, beyond or before the moment of conception. At what point does memory begin? And what is the reach of recall? That is an interesting question to wrestle with.

Do you think then, just furthering the conversation, that the way arts therapies have developed veers more towards one or the other of those memories? Do you think there is a tendency towards more explicit work, in terms of memories that we can recall from our personal histories and testimonies?

Aleka Loutsis: I think it can go both ways, I really do. Sometimes there is a current narrative, an explicit memory of something a person has experienced in their life. There could also be implicit echoes of a generational narrative in the background, what you inherit from your family, the cultural memory of the family. So, there is the current narrative, whatever that is, which is the explicit memory. But then if you are working creatively through the artform, other motifs can emerge spontaneously through the movement, other shapes, patterns of movement, which may not be familiar. Sometimes, the embodied expression is directly related to the current narrative, but other times something more surprising emerges, something unknown rises up from the shadows. I was just thinking how this can also occur across different cultures. It reminds me of some recent group therapy work, where the overarching theme was of grief, relating to loss, violence and death. What arose was the creation of a sculpt using various props and spontaneous body movements, one of which was the action of tearing paper. In that moment the sculpt was animated with an embodied expression of feeling and as an act of remembrance. For some cultures, such as in the Jewish community, the tearing of the cloth is symbolic of loss and grief, following the death of a loved one. That is just one example, but you could have prayer motifs or despairing gestures, there are many movement motifs that come. So, in this example, we can consider the extent to which both the personal and the collective experience of grief may have been expressed through the artform.

Richard Hougham: Coming back to the example that you gave of your clinical practice where motifs can emerge which are a kind of echo of an aspect of a cultural practice – in this case the idea of tearing as part of a grief ritual. That questioning of where the implicit memory comes from is an interesting one. It reminds me of Jung talking about one of the first moments he thought about the idea of the collective unconscious, when he was working in New York in 1913. A schizophrenic patient took him to the window and described a vision of the sun and said to Jung something along the lines of, "If you look at the sun, there is a tube of wind and it's the origin of the wind. You can see the tube of the wind underneath the sun and then if you move your head to the left then the sun goes with you, and then if you move your head to the right then the sun will also move with you." This was relatively early on in Jung's professional life as a doctor and he thought it was a delusion, a psychosis which didn't mean anything. Then four years later he came across a previously unpublished manuscript on Egyptian mythology, which referred to an Egyptian myth which told the story of the origin of the wind being a tube which came down from the sun, and also if you move your head to the left and then to the right, so the sun goes with you. It was a description of the vision of this patient, who would not have been able to have seen this particular transcript. Jung said that was his first hint towards something of a collective unconscious, which seems pertinent to this conversation in terms of memory. So, I wondered, especially working in mental health, how do we as practitioners respond to memories and motifs? It strikes me that the way you are responding to the tearing was trying to understand it symbolically and culturally, or as an artistic practice.

Aleka Loutsis: So, we brought these two forms of memory together, that was the thing. Or the one brought out the other, I mean they are interrelated.

Richard Hougham: The implicit and the explicit, they are co-existent, it is not a binary.

Aleka Loutsis: That's right. Explicit memory forms later, after implicit memory. But then we have both. And I like that, I like the fact that there is the possibility of working in both ways. Of course, it is important to note that when there has been severe trauma in the frame then we are dealing with a much more vulnerable and fragmented system, which inevitably will influence our approach.

Richard Hougham: Are there other terms for it?

Aleka Loutsis: To me it parallels the unconscious and conscious, from a Jungian point of view. Actually, we could also think about it in terms of bottom-up and top-down processes, which have influenced my work on the gestures in terms of repairing missing developmental experiences or retrieving lost parts of self (Loutsis, in Hougham and Jones, 2017, p. 149).

Richard Hougham: But explicit suggests that you can recall something. You might not necessarily be conscious of it in the moment, but I can think to myself, "I'm going to ask myself the question," or "I am going to take myself back to my childhood home," or "I am going to take myself back to a particular moment in my own history," and then there is a capacity I have to recall something, that would be more explicit.

Aleka Loutsis: Yes, that is how I would understand it. Whereas working spontaneously with movement, perhaps with the intention that you remain curious as to what might come up, then you may receive some new information. You might still recall a memory, but also there is a possibility of something other emerging when you are working in the unconscious field.

Richard Hougham: It is also a question of the self and whether the self is created from the moment that we were born or whether we have a predisposition which carries some sort of memory. So, we are back to ancestral memory or back to double memory or back to implicit memory.

So, I'd like to ask a question about your work with developmental gestures, which is something I know you have been working on for the past few years. I mean, there is a very clear outline of these gestures in terms of what they evoke and what they can elicit in terms of memory. So, talk me through your thinking about the developmental gestures and how they relate to questions of memory.

Aleka Loutsis: The five actions of yield, push, reach, grasp and pull originate from research Bonnie Bainbridge Cohen (1993) carried out on patterns of movement during infant development which were part of a much wider and in-depth analysis of human movement and the intelligence of the body. These developmental gestures are universal actions or movements that are originally formed within the primary relationship during infancy but that can also be observed throughout our lives. In our infancy, these developmental actions perform an important function, forming an attachment with our caregivers and getting our needs met in order to survive. We are looking at those first experiences of yielding to being held, having the desire to reach towards something, needing to push to be able to reach and take hold of that something and then pull it back in towards you. This cycle of yielding, pushing, reaching, grasping and pulling can be seen as a framework within which the developing child learns about their relationship to another, to an object or to an idea. What's important here, in terms of memory, is how those demands are met because the quality of attention, care and response to those needs, form embodied and embedded patterns of behaviour and belief systems that stay with us in adulthood and can be played out in many aspects of our lives. For example, if we had repeatedly unhelpful responses to reaching out, then later on in life the meaning-making around that will be, "If I reach out, I don't get what I need so I will just deal with it myself."

Richard Hougham: So, our memories of those inform our later relationship with other people in the world. I guess what follows on from that is the opportunity within dance movement therapy and drama and movement therapy to reckon with those and pivot those and explore and be curious about different gestures and rehearsing new ways of relating.

Aleka Loutsis: Exactly, so, first of all, studying them and noticing how one – I am just going to use reach as an example – how one reaches. Whether you are reaching with the top of your hand or whether you are reaching with your palm up. How far does your arm reach out? Where does the reach begin in your body? Really taking time to study the action of reaching in detail. It's very hard to reach out when this action hasn't been seen and responded to; some people really struggle to even move their arm and it's as simple as that. Some people will just keep their arm by their side. So, the work becomes about re-learning this basic developmental gesture and creatively exploring different ways of getting to know it. But there must be a generational element to this too. Certain relational ways of being are passed on from one generation to the next and so we inherit an embodied lineage that has been formed across time.

Richard Hougham: Like a family legacy of something which has either been developed and enhanced or neglected or arrested?

Aleka Loutsis: Exactly, and you can look at that in terms of emotions, some families won't accept anger, or others won't accept sadness, some emotions are just less well tolerated than others. In my mind it's a similar idea.

Richard Hougham: That is really interesting in terms of those developmental gestures, and would you mind talking us through the gestures again?

Aleka Loutsis: They begin with yielding; think of an infant being held and supported in their parents' arms. There is a relational and an active quality to this interaction, it is not passive. Imagine the infant on their hands and knees, swinging back and forth, discovering the push they need to mobilise their body towards something they need or want. Then, using that push to reach out and grasp that object and bring it back in towards them (Loutsis, A. in Hougham and Jones (eds.), 2017, p. 150).

Richard Hougham: And then that's the cycle and then they fall on their bottom again!

Aleka Loutsis: Yes! And yielding is the most important action because it requires trust, which is fundamental to everything. Certainly, if we are thinking about how we might access less conscious memories, then we need to be able to yield (Loutsis in Hougham and Jones (eds.), 2021, p. 86).

Richard Hougham: Again, it reminds me of analytical psychology in terms of how Jung's work suggested that we need to find ways to lend an ear to the unconscious and not to fix ourselves too much with the limited and rather narrow view of the ego. But of course, that it is easier said than done in terms of letting go, and I think that letting go, whether that being to sleep or whether that being to a place of not knowing, letting go of some sort of control over things, is a similar quality to yielding. But then if the ground hasn't been there for you before, then you might not have the trust to be able to feel like you are going to land safely. So, it is an interesting dynamic of trying to think about where, as an arts therapist, to begin with yielding. Perhaps foundations and the floor?

Aleka Loutsis: Absolutely, and of course with movement, the floor, the ground is vital both for landing safely and also for taking off into unknown territory. But I was thinking about that idea of letting go, and going back to what you said just before, whether listening is a more helpful way of engaging that idea through the body. So, paying attention and listening to what is happening inside and not be so preoccupied with the letting go, because that can be a block.

Richard Hougham: Right, that pressure on yourself to let go is just the antithesis of letting go.

Aleka Loutsis: Yeah, immediately you are tensing up. So, I really like that idea of paying attention, listen and follow, see, feel, sense what is going on inside and not have an agenda.

Richard Hougham: That kind of reminds me of the idea of bearing witness to something rather than ploughing through with agenda supposition or an ideology, but actually how challenging it can be to bear witness.

Aleka Loutsis: It was Joan Chodorow (1991, p. 112) who said when discussing movement in relation to active imagination, that the body grounds the limitlessness of the unconscious. We have a material body, so however deeply we dive or however high we fly, whichever dimension you follow, the body, at some level is going to keep you grounded and that's an interesting concept. The idea that you have a material body but also a subtle body is one that has also inspired my work on yielding into the "dreamdance," where the experience is beyond real time while remaining grounded in our physical body (Loutsis, in Hougham and Jones, 2021, p. 86). When describing the subtle body, Arnold Mindell (1982) tells us that it can be expressed in different ways such as through dream images when asleep or spontaneously when "the dancer experiences the "dreambody" as the creative impulse behind movement" (p. 51).

Richard Hougham: Like, the body is there as the housing. Which I guess prompts the question in terms of serious mental health conditions and disassociation, there's a gulf between those two things. There is no anchor point for some of those psychological experiences.

Aleka Loutsis: Yeah, and that's why sometimes you have to work in a more concrete, conscious or explicit way with movement and the body, towards a more integrated and coherent state of the whole system.

Richard Hougham: I've got one more question, just because we are coming to the end of the conversation. As an artist, and your background is in dance, you have been working for many years as a teacher and arts therapy practitioner, I was wondering are there any artists that you have seen over the years that have inspired you in thinking about this theme of memory, thinking about shaping memories? I was just wondering if you can recall, maybe a particular show or experience you had?

Aleka Loutsis: The image that came up as you posed the question was of my first experience of going to the theatre when I was very young and seeing a classical ballet; it was a Russian ballet company, and the ballet was Giselle, a romantic ballet. It just captivated me completely. The beauty of bodies moving gracefully in space and the clarity of lines, geometric lines, but also the transporting sense of a spiritual dimension or some other dimension which had the power to transcend a story of betrayal and end with the redemptive power of love. It goes back to what we were saying about the material body and the experience of something closer to the dream world. It is interesting that you ask this question, because I think my passion for movement in all its dimensions probably stems from that one moment.

Richard Hougham: It is interesting that you mentioned geometric shapes, so the form in the space linking to something that is of a different order. The question of shaping which is part of the conversation of how you shape memories and the relationship between form and non-form. I mean in that case it was form.

Aleka Loutsis: But it is also non-form, that is the thing. There is something about the form, when we have understood and mastered it, that enables the form to dissolve. So, I think if we can be disciplined in the form, whatever form it is, in that case it was classical ballet, but there is no reason why discipline can't be applied to listening to what is happening inside the body as it moves in the space.

Richard Hougham: This is a really nice place to end, the philosophy of form reminds me of structure and anti-structure in Victor Turner's work in terms of the ritual process – without the structure, the container of the ritual, then you won't have the transformational qualities within it. The relationship between form and non-form is a profound one.

Aleka Loutsis: It is, and the relationship between the body moving in space, space inside body, space around body, how the shapes are created in the space, all the dimensions of space seen and unseen, play an important part of what we have been talking about.

Richard Hougham: Thank you very much.

References

Chodorow, J. (1991). *Dance Therapy & Depth Psychology: The Moving Imagination*. London: Routledge.

Cohen, B.B. (1993). *Sensing, Feeling, and Action: The Experiential Anatomy of Body-Mind Centering*. Northampton, MA: Contact Editions.

Dunlea, M. (2019). *BodyDreaming in the Treatment of Developmental Trauma*. Oxford: Routledge.

Gerhardt, S, (2004). *Why Love Matters: How Affection Shapes a Baby's Brain*. Hove: Brunner-Routledge.

Hougham, R. and Jones, B. (eds.). (2017). *Dramatherapy. Reflections and Praxis*. London: Palgrave.

Hougham, R. smd Jones, B. (eds.). (2021). *Dramatherapy. The Nature of Interruption*. Oxon: Routledge.

Mindell, A. (1982). *Dreambody: The Body's Role in Revealing the Self*. London: Arkana Penguin Books.

Ogden, P., Minton, K., and Pain, C. (2006). *Trauma and the Body: A Sensorimotor Approach to Psychotherapy*. London and New York: W.W. Norton & Co.

Porges, S. (2011). *The Polyvagal Theory: Neurophysiological Foundations of Emotions, Attachment, Communication, Self-Regulation*. New York: W.W. Norton & Co.

Van der Kolk, B. (2014). *The Body Keeps the Score: Mind, Brain and Body in the Transformation of Trauma*. London: Allen Lane Penguin Books.

BIOGRAPHIES

Editors

Marián Cao, PhD, is Professor and Chair of Art Education and Art Therapy at the University Complutense of Madrid, Spain. She was the founding director of the university's Art Therapy masters programme and formerly the director of the PhD programme on Art, Art Therapy and Social Inclusion. She has coordinated several Latinoamerican university programmes. Marián has published several books on women and art, art therapy and trauma and the social functions of art. She is the main researcher of the national project BRUNDIBÁR: Art therapy as a path for wellbeing in the face of childhood trauma. Marián has directed several national and European research projects, including DiverCity ("diving into diversity in museums and in the city"), ARIADNE (Art and Intercultural integration), POWER and MUSYGEN on gender and museums. She is a member of the committee of experts in culture of the Organization of Ibero-American States for Education, Science and Culture (OEI).

Richard Hougham, MA, is a Principal Lecturer and Course Leader of the MA in Drama and Movement Therapy at the Royal Central School of Speech and Drama, University of London, England. He has a special interest in storytelling and the language of myth as part of the Sesame approach to dramatherapy and as a teaching pedagogy. He is currently Chair of the European Consortium of Arts Therapies Education (ECArTE). Richard continues to develop his interest in the connections between analytical psychology and the arts. His current research is an enquiry into storytelling of myth and fairytale in the training of the dramatherapist.

Sarah Scoble, MA, is Honorary President of the European Consortium of Arts Therapies Education (ECArTE) and Series Editor with Professor Diane Waller for the annual *International Research in the Arts Therapies* publication with Routledge, in association with ECArTE and the International Centre for Research in Arts Therapies (ICRA). She served on the Executive Board of ECArTE for many years and was Chair from 2009 to 2017. Formerly, Head of the Centre for Performing Arts and Media at South Devon College, UK, where she was also a founder trainer of the UK's first southwest postgraduate Diploma in Dramatherapy. Later, Course Leader of the Exeter-based Masters in Dramatherapy programmes and Director of the Southwest School for Dramatherapy Limited. She has edited many ECArTE publications and has a developing interest in the use of the arts and the imagination in the management of chronic pain.

Chapter authors

Karima Anbar, MA, is a French diplomat, who has extensive expertise working in human rights, women's rights, political analysis and civil societies in Arab countries. After completing her Masters in Political Sciences at the Institute of Political Sciences in Lyon, she started her career working for French Foreign Ministry for eight years in Arab countries such as Jordan, Palestine, UAE and Kuwait. Ms Karima also worked closely with high profile individuals, international organisations and institutions. Last but not least, she is renowned for her remarkably strong advocacy for women's rights and human rights.

Recent publications include:

Sakhi, S., Kreidie, L., Wardani, F., Anbar, K. and AlSabah, I. (2022). Drama therapy as a mental health intervention for women in the shatila refugee camp, Lebanon. *Intervention*, 20(1), 58. https://doi.org/10.4103/intv.intv_12_20.

Sakhi, S., Kreidie, L., Wardani, F., AlSabah, I. and Anbar, K. (2020). The power of theater expression and communication: A psychological therapeutic intervention in a refugee camp: An IPA Study into the Narratives of Women Refugees' Experience With Drama Therapy. *Psychology Research*, 10(1), 10–23. doi: 10.17265/2159-5542/2020.01.002.

Orcid-ID: 0009-0000-4701-9006

Audronė Brazauskaitė, PhD (social sciences: educology (07 S), Vilnius Pedagogical University, 2001). This was the first time in Lithuania that a thesis was defended based on art therapy for children with learning disabilities – *Developing a Sense of Self Through Art in Children with Severe and Moderate Learning Disabilities*. Audronė is an art therapist and a pioneer of this profession in Lithuania, supervisor and founder member of the Lithuanian Art

Therapy Association. She has worked in the interdepartmental work groups, aiming at the formalisation of art therapy as a profession in Lithuania. Audronė has been part of the work group which created Lithuania's first second-level joint programme in art therapy at the Lithuanian University of Health Sciences (LSMU) – Vilnius Academy of Arts (VDA). She is a lecturer at the Vilnius University Medical Faculty. Founder and director of the Public Enterprise Arts Therapy Centre. Research areas: art therapy, image perception, visual creation, interdisciplinary discourse.

Recent publications include:

Tautkevičius, V. and Brazauskaitė, A. (2018). Epilepsija sergančiųjų potyriai dailės terapijos metu. Experiences of people with epilepsy during art therapy. *Rehabilitation Sciences: Nursing, Physiotherapy, Ergotherapy*; *Lithuanian Sports University Klaipeda University*, 1(18) 2018 ISSN 2029–3194 / eISSN 2538–8673, https://www.researchgate.net/publication/333138895_EPILEPSIJA_SERGANCIUJU_POTYRIAI_DAILES_TERAPIJOS_METU.

Brazauskaitė, A. (2017). Garsiai kalbantys piešiniai [Drawings speeking out loud]. In S. Mostauskis and A. Brazauskaitė (ed), *Menas, terapija, sveikata* [*Art, Therapy, Health*]. Kaunas: Lietuvos sveikatos mokslų universiteto Leidybos namai.

Brazauskaitė, A. and Dikčiūtė, S. (2015). *Modernaus meno socialinė reikšmė: meniniai socialiniai performansai* [*Social Aspect of Modern Art: performances*]. Menų terapijos centras.

Orcid-ID: 0009-0003-0449-3121

Marián Cao, PhD, is an art therapist and University Professor at University Complutense of Madrid. Marián has had long academic stays in Germany (Akademie der Künste, Munich and Hochschüle der Künste, Berlin), the UK (Courtald Institute of Art, London), the USA (MOMA, New York) and Mexico (University of Veracruz). She is currently Director of the consolidated research group EARTDI 941035: Applications of art in social inclusion (https://www.ucm.es/eartdi); Vice-chair, since 2017, of the European Consortium of Arts Therapies Education (https://www.ecarte.info/); and Member of the committee of experts in culture of the Organization of Ibero-American States for Education, Science and Culture (OEI).

Recent publications include:

López Fernández Cao, M. (2023). The Artist's Book as a Form of Autoethnography for the Teaching Profession. In A. Bautista García-Vera, *Photographic Elicitation and Narration in Teachers Education and Development*. Switzerland, Springer. https://doi.org/10.1007/978-3-031-20164-6.

López-Escribano, Orío-Aparicio, C. and López Fernández Cao, M. (2023). An overview of historical and contemporary perspectives in art therapy in Spain: A bibliometric analysis of Spanish art therapy research. *The Arts in Psychotherapy*, 83, 102015. https://doi.org/10.1016/j.aip.2023.102015.

López Fernández Cao, M. (2021). On the unknown that art addresses: Space, vacuum and awareness in the arts. In M. López Fernández Cao, R. Hougham and S. Scoble, *Imagining Windmills: Trust, Truth and the Unknown in Arts Therapies*. London: Routledge.

Orcid-ID: 0000-0003-0421-3612

Alanah Garrard, MA, is a UKCP registered existential psychotherapist and supervisor and has a private practice in West London. She trained in 2000 as a drama and movement therapist, and later went on to an MA in Integrative Therapy and an Advanced Diploma in Existential Therapy. In addition to her private practice, she teaches developmental psychology and performing research on the MA Drama and Movement Therapy course at the Royal Central School of Speech and Drama, as well as offering clinical supervision to the students in their second year of training. Her areas of research include unspoken communication within the therapeutic relationship and the role developmental psychology plays in our developing sense of self and relationships.

Recent publications include:

Garrard, A. (2021). Image of the mind's eye. In R. Hougham and B. Jones (eds), *Dramatherapy: The Nature of Interruption*. Oxford: Routledge.

Garrard, A. (2017). The Gaze. In R. Hougham and B. Jones (eds), *Dramatherapy: Reflections and Praxis*. London: Red Globe Press.

Joy Gravestock, PhD, is a violinist, music therapist, supervisor and lecturer. She works in the East Midlands, within the adoption community, and brings lived experience to her professional life. She previously sat on both Nottingham and Leicester Adoption Panels as an Independent Member. Currently she is an identified specialist therapist for adoptees and their families within Leicester County/City and works with other Midlands local authorities, as well as independently with major national and local adoption charities. Her PhD at Sheffield University explored adoption, the neurobiology of attachment and the efficacy of psychoanalytic music therapy as a reparative therapy especially with regard to attunement. She is passionate about advocating for appropriate services that are shaped by the expressed needs of the adoption community and works to ensure music therapists are able to dictate adequate therapeutic resources for adoptees. Additionally, Joy is a senior lecturer on the MA Music Therapy training at the University of Western England.

Recent publications include:

Gravestock, J. (2022). Micro moments of attunement with an adopted child: A single case study of intersubjective music therapy, with implications for the practice of music therapy enabling reparation of familial difficulties, within the adoption community. PhD thesis, University of Sheffield. Available as a free download at the White Rose Repository. See https://etheses.whiterose.ac.uk.

Gravestock, J. (2019). Psychoanalytic relational music therapy for children with high-functioning autism in specialist school placements. In H. Dunn, E. Coombes, E. Maclean, H. Mottram and J. Nugent (Eds), *Music Therapy and Autism: A Spectrum of Approaches*. London: Jessica Kingsley Publishers.

Gravestock, J. (2018). Attachment-based, relational, psychoanalytic music therapy: the significance of musical moments of attunement with adoptees after trauma, and how this may influence broader reparation with attachments. *Attachment: New Directions in Psychotherapy and Relational Psychoanalysis*, 12(2), 147–159.

Vera Heller, PhD, is Professor of Art Therapy at the University of Québec in Abitibi – Témiscamingue (UQAT) in Montréal, a psychotherapist and fine artist. Having studied in social work, fine arts and art therapy, she obtained her PhD from Lesley University. Vera taught in Brazil, Japan, and Thailand and facilitated workshops in Quebec, Cuba and Mexico. Along with her artistic practice, these art therapy-based activities inspired her research projects about displacement issues, narrative identity and artistic creation. Her research projects consist of explorations of lived experiences from a variety of perspectives. Most often, they include both the artistic and the psychotherapeutic components of art therapy. Vera's latest project, titled *My Life, an Artist's Book*, took place at the Montreal Museum of Fine Arts. It explores the life stories of a group of immigrant co-researchers from an autoethnographic and artistic perspective.

Recent publications include:

Heller, V. (2023). Le parcours du Héros: Une intervention de groupe auprès des migrants existentiels [The Hero's journey: A group intervention with existential migrants]. In L. Pelletier and J. Lambert (eds.), *L'art-thérapie auprès des groupes: Réflexions théoriques et développements cliniques*. Quebec: PUQ.

Heller, V. (2023). Qu'y a-t-il derrière le masque de la morale prolétarienne qui me réduit au silence? [What is behind the mask of proletarian morality that silences me?]. *International Journal Sociocultural Community Development and Practices*, UQAM, Vol. 25 (June 2024). https://edition.uqam.ca/atps/article/view/1542.

Heller, V. (2007). Exile, identity, and artistic creation: An arts-based phenomenological study with immigrant women. Doctoral dissertation, Lesley University. https://digitalcommons.lesley.edu/expressive_dissertations/33/.

Orcid-ID: 0000-0002-6339-0371

HH Sheikha Intisar AlSabah, BA, is a Kuwaiti social entrepreneur, philanthropist, author, film producer and columnist whose vision is of a peaceful and aspirational Arab world. Her humanitarian work, philanthropic and entrepreneurial initiatives have become even more significant in scope, reach and impact. Her Highness launched a pioneering initiative to heal one million Arabs through the use of dramatherapy after establishing Intisar Foundation. In 2018, HH Sheikha Intisar AlSabah started the process of launching Intisar Foundation, a UK registered charity dedicated to supporting Arab women affected by war through the creative and therapeutic approach of dramatherapy. The Foundation was officially registered with the UK and Wales Charity Commission on 8 March, 2019, marking International Women's Day. It is the first organisation to work on the mental health of women affected by war and trauma in the Arab world.

Recent publications include:

Sakhi, S., Kreidie, L., Wardani, F., Anbar, K. and AlSabah, I. (2022). Drama therapy as a mental health intervention for women in the shatila refugee camp, Lebanon. *Intervention*, 20(1), 58. https://doi.org/10.4103/intv.intv_12_20.

Sakhi, S., Kreidie, L., Wardani, F., AlSabah, I. and Anbar, K. (2020). The power of theater expression and communication: A psychological therapeutic intervention in a refugee camp: An IPA Study Into the Narratives of Women Refugees' Experience with Drama Therapy. *Psychology Research*, 10(1), 10–23. doi: 10.17265/2159-5542/2020.01.002.

Orcid-ID: 0009-0008-8966-0836

Lina Haddad Kreidie, PhD, is the Academic Director of the TLS-gender programme at the Lebanese American University (LAU). Kreidie is a political psychologist, an assistant professor and a research consultant on Women's Empowerment at Intisar Foundation. Kreidie is also a 2018 US Fulbright Scholar, a Jerome and Hazel Tobis fellow at the University of California, Irvine Interdisciplinary Center for the Scientific Study of Ethics and Morality, a member of the Harris Council University of Chicago Harris School for Public Policy, joining its council for public policy between 2012 and 2022, and an affiliate faculty at the Pearson institute for the study and resolution of conflict at the University of Chicago.

Recent publications include:

Kreidie, L.H., Kreidie, M. and Atassi, H. (2016). Living with ongoing political trauma: The prevalence and impact of PTSD among Syrian refugees. *Journal of Psychology Research*, 6(10). https://doi.org/10.17265/2159-5542/2016.10.005

Kreidie, L.H. and Monroe, K.R. (2002). Psychological boundaries and ethnic conflict: How identity constrained choice and worked to turn ordinary people into perpetrators of ethnic violence during the Lebanese civil war. *International Journal of Politics, Culture and Society*, 16(1), 5–36. https://doi.org/10.1023/a:1016578210778

Sakhi, S., Kreidie, L., Wardani, F., Anbar, K. and AlSabah, I. (2022). Drama therapy as a mental health intervention for women in the Shatila refugee camp, Lebanon. *Intervention*, 20(1), 58. https://doi.org/10.4103/intv.intv_12_20.

Sakhi, S., Kreidie, L., Wardani, F., AlSabah, I. and Anbar, K. (2020). The power of theater expression and communication: A psychological therapeutic intervention in a refugee camp: An IPA Study Into the Narratives of Women Refugees' Experience with Drama Therapy. *Psychology Research*, 10(1), 10–23. doi: 10.17265/2159-5542/2020.01.002.

Orcid-ID: 0000-0001-6617-1951

Aleka Loutsis, MA, is a dramatherapist and dance movement psychotherapist. She teaches movement on the MA Drama & Movement Therapy Course at the Royal Central School of Speech and Drama, University of London. Aleka works for the National Health Service in adult mental health within Secondary Care Specialist Psychological Services. She has a private practice in therapy and supervision and actively promotes an embodied approach, drawing upon her clinical and research experience and her specialist training in the treatment of complex trauma. Her particular interest is in working creatively with the body and movement to alleviate the impact of trauma. Aleka has guest lectured on other therapy trainings nationally and internationally and has facilitated movement workshops for the ECArTE conferences.

Recent publications include:

Loutsis, A. (2021). Dreamdance. In R. Hougham and B. Jones (ed.), *Dramatherapy: The Nature of Interruption*. Oxford: Routledge.

Loutsis, A. (2017). Body, movement and trauma. In R. Hougham and B. Jones (ed.), *Dramatherapy: Reflections and Praxis*. London: Palgrave.

Unnur Óttarsdóttir, PhD, has practised art therapy in private practice and in a variety of organisations, including schools, for over three decades. She has taught art therapy at the Iceland University of the Arts, the continuing education department of the University of Akureyri, the British Association of Art Therapists, the Art Therapy Association of Romania, the University of Hertfordshire and Art Therapy Italiana. Unnur is a researcher at the Reykjavik Academy. She has written articles and book chapters about art therapy in education, memory drawing and the methodology of grounded theory. Her research interests include art therapy in education for children who have experienced trauma and have specific learning difficulties, as well as art making as a therapeutic and learning approach. Unnur has given lectures on these topics in Iceland and worldwide.

Recent publications include:

Óttarsdóttir, U. (2019). Ethical concern when applying Drawing for Memory: Research Conducted in Iceland. In: A. Di Maria (Ed.). *Exploring Ethical Dilemmas in Art Therapy: 50 Clinicians From 20 Countries Share Their Stories* (pp. 266–272). New York, Routledge.

Óttarsdóttir, U. (2018). Processing Emotions and Memorising Coursework through Memory Drawing. *ATOL: Art Therapy OnLine*, 9(1).

Óttarsdóttir, U. (2010). Art Therapy in Education for Children with Specific Learning Difficulties Who Have Experienced Stress and/or Trauma. In: V. Karkou (Ed.), *Arts Therapies in Schools: Research and Practice* (pp. 145–160). London, Jessica Kingsley Publishers.

Orcid-ID 0000-0002-2438-7233

Eha Rüütel, PhD, in psychology, Master of Public Health, is a registered solution-focused psychotherapist, creative arts therapist (art therapy) and supervisor. Currently working as a Distinguished Professor of Creative Arts Therapies at the School of Natural Sciences and Health of Tallinn University, Estonia. The representative of Tallinn University in the European Consortium for Arts Therapies Education (ECArTE). Founder and honorary member of the Estonian Association of Creative Arts Therapies. Art therapy practice with adults and adolescents with mental health challenges. As the initiator of the arts therapies' specialty at Tallinn University and a member of the occupational committee at the Estonian Qualifications Authority, Eha has been involved in development of the concept of arts therapies and qualification requirements for therapists. Current research and teaching are mainly concerned with behavioural correlates of health, application of a solution-focused approach to art therapy and self-development, application of the arts in the school context.

Recent publications include:

Krüger, V., Macedo, E., Addessi, A.R., Rüütel, E., Warner, C., Carvalho, A. and Bunt, L. (2020). Learning how to learn: The role of music and other expressive arts in responding to Early Leaving from Education and Training

(ELET) in the STALWARTS project. *Voices: A World Forum for Music Therapy*, 20(3), 17. https://doi.org/10.15845/voices.v20i3.3084.

Rüütel, E., Kruus, K., Ivanova, A. and Laas, K. (2018). Structured short-term group art therapy for patients with fibromyalgia. A pilot study. *Journal of Rehabilitation Sciences: Nursing, Physiotherapy, Ergotherapy*, 18(1), 42–52. https://doi.org/10.33607/rmske.v1i18.753.

Rüütel, E. (2017). Loovteraapia kontseptsioonist, rakendamisest ja tõenduspõhisusest [The concept, implementation and evidence base of creative arts therapy]. *Eesti Arst, 96*(11), 661–668. https://eestiarst.ee/loovteraapia-kontseptsioonist-rakendamisest-ja-toenduspohisusest/.

Orcid-ID: 0000-0001-7698-5377

Nisha Sajnani, PhD, is an Associate Professor and Director of the NYU Program in Drama Therapy and the chair of the NYU Creative Arts Therapies Consortium. She is the founding co-director of the Jameel Arts & Health Lab, established in collaboration with the World Health Organisation (WHO), where she leads the Lancet global series on the health benefits of the arts. Nisha received her PhD in interdisciplinary studies, combining drama therapy and community economic development, from the School of Community and Public Affairs at Concordia University in Montreal. An award-winning author, educator and advocate, her body of work explores unique ways in which aesthetic experience can inspire equity, care and collective human flourishing across the lifespan.

Recent publications include:

Dokter, D. and Sajnani, N. (2023) *Intercultural Dramatherapy: Imagination and Action at the Intersection of Difference*. Oxford: Routledge.

Sajnani, N. and Fietje, N. (2023). The Jameel Arts & Health Lab – Lancet series on the health benefits of the arts, in collaboration with the WHO. *The Lancet*. doi.org/10.1016/S0140-6736(23)01959-1.

Sajnani, N., Willemsen, M., and Butler, J. (2023). Scoping review on the observed benefits of Developmental Transformations. *Drama Therapy Review*, 9(2), 273–315. doi.org/10.1386/dtr_00133_1.

Orcid-ID: 0000-0001-5805-6179

Sara Sakhi, BSc, is a researcher who works directly with war-affected women receiving dramatherapy-based psychological interventions in Lebanon. She has conducted both quantitative and qualitative research over the course of three years with Intisar Foundation. Sakhi is adamant on the importance of providing sound scientific evidence of the importance of psychological support for war-affected populations, especially in war-torn Arab countries. She is currently completeing her Masters in Social Work and Human Rights.

Recent publications include:

Sakhi, S., Kreidie, L., Wardani, F., Anbar, K. and AlSabah, I. (2022). Drama therapy as a mental health intervention for women in the Shatila refugee camp, Lebanon. *Intervention*, 20(1), 58. https://doi.org/10.4103/intv.intv_12_20.

Sakhi, S., Kreidie, L., Wardani, F., AlSabah, I. and Anbar, K. (2020). The power of theater expression and communication: A psychological therapeutic intervention in a refugee camp: An IPA Study Into the Narratives of Women Refugees' Experience with Drama Therapy. *Psychology Research*, 10(1), 10–23. doi: 10.17265/2159-5542/2020.01.002.

Orcid-ID: 0000-0002-0116-8046

Gabriele Schmid, PhD, studied Fine Art and Art Education at the University of Arts in Berlin. From 2004–2007 she held a deputy professorship at the Carl von Ossietzky Universität Oldenburg for Art Education – visual culture and its didactic. Since 2007 she has been Professor for Aesthetic Education at the Hochschule für Künste im Sozialen, Ottersberg (University of Applied Sciences and Arts, Ottersberg). Since 2015 she has been academic principal for research, studies and teaching at the HKS Ottersberg. From 2015 to 2022 Gabriele was part of the executive board of the Society of Artistic Research. Her research interests are in the fields of arts-based and artistic research with a specialisation in artistic autoethnography. As an artist she is working in the fields of sculpting, drawing and installation.

Recent publications include:

Schulze-Stampa, C. and Schmid, G. (2022). Kollaboration, interaktion und partizipation in künstlerischen und künstlerisch-therapeutischen prozessen. In P. Bettzieche and U. Apolte (eds.), *Kaleidoskop. Vielfalt kunsttherapeutischer Interventionen*. Lengerich: Pabst Science Publishers.

Schulze-Stampa, C. and Schmid, G. (eds.) (2020). *Kunst im Krankenhaus: Interdisziplinäre Zusammenarbeit und Perspektivwechsel in Gesundheitsförderung und Prävention*. Stuttgart: Kohlhammer.

Schmid, G. (2020). After images: Participatory observation as artistic autoethnography. In G. Schmid *et al.* (eds.), *Teilnehmende Beobachtung in den künstlerischen Therapien. Band 8 der Reihe Wissenschaftliche Grundlagen der Künstlerischen Therapien*. Berlin: HBP University Press.

Orcid-ID: 0000-0001-6950-7684

Raquel Chapin Stephenson, PhD, ATR-BC, LCAT, is a Professor of Art Therapy at Lesley University. She is also Adjunct Faculty at the School of Visual Arts. As a Fulbright Scholar, she taught at Tallinn University in Estonia and continues as a guest lecturer. She recently published the book *Art Therapy and Creative*

Aging: Reclaiming Elderhood, Health and Wellbeing. She was co-founder and teaching artist for the Creative Approaches to Healthy Aging programme, funded by two NEA ArtWorks Grants, and founded New York University's Creative Aging Therapeutic Services. She serves on the National Advisory Council of Arts for the Aging, the Advisory Council for First Aid of the Soul: Psychosocial Support for Ukraine, and the Advisory Council of the Art Therapy Project, and is a member of the UNESCO-UNITWIN Chair on Life Design, Decent Work and Sustainable Development.

Recent publications include:

Stephenson, R.C. (2021). *Art Therapy and Creative Aging: Reclaiming Elderhood, Health and Wellbeing*. New York: Routledge.

Orcid-ID: 0000-0002-0177-0969

Farah Wardani, MA, is a Lebanese theatre actress, trainer, clown doctor, puppeteer and applied theatre practitioner. Farah is a theatre graduate with an MA in Dramatherapy, a Diploma of High Studies in Theatre and a BA in Psychology. She is a Playback Theatre practitioner, trainer, actress and conductor. A director of Laban, a Lebanese theatre-based NGO that uses social and psychosocial theatre approaches for social change, capacity building and therapy. She leads dramatherapy workshops with the Intisar Foundation engaging with Arab women affected of war and violence. Farah trains and uses Theater of the Oppressed, Dramatherapy and other techniques with different communities and contexts as a medium for healing, social change and political activism.

Recent publications include:

R Sakhi, S., Kreidie, L., Wardani, F., Anbar, K. and AlSabah, I. (2022). Drama therapy as a mental health intervention for women in the Shatila refugee camp, Lebanon. *Intervention*, 20(1), 58. https://doi.org/10.4103/intv.intv_12_20.

Sakhi, S., Kreidie, L., Wardani, F., AlSabah, I. and Anbar, K. (2020). The power of theater expression and communication: A psychological therapeutic intervention in a refugee camp: An IPA Study Into the Narratives of Women Refugees' Experience with Drama Therapy. *Psychology Research*, 10(1), 10–23. doi: 10.17265/2159-5542/2020.01.002.

Orcid-ID: 0009-0005-4474-1411

Printed and bound by CPI Group (UK) Ltd, Croydon, CR0 4YY
20/08/2024
01027706-0006